AT LAST!

EVERYTHING YOU EVER NEEDED TO KNOW ABOUT

ALLERGIES . . . ARTHRITIS . . . BACKACHE . . . BEDWETTING . . . BLOOD PRESSURE . . . BUR-SITIS . . . CHOLESTEROL . . . CONSTIPATION . . . DENTAL PROBLEMS . . . DIZZY SPELLS . . . EYE PROBLEMS . . . ESTROGEN . . . FACIAL HAIR . . . FAILING MEMORY . . . HERNIA . . . HIGH BLOOD SUGAR . . . IMPOTENCE . . . MENOPAUSE . . . MYASTHENIA GRAVIS . . . NEURITIS . . . NOSE-BLEEDS . . . OBESITY . . . PHLEBITIS . . . THE PILL . . . PROSTATE . . . SINUSITIS . . . STROKE . . . ULCERS . . . VAGINAL INFECTION . . . VARI-COSE VEINS . . . VITAMIN POISONING . . . WHIP-LASH, AND MUCH, MUCH MORE.

> *Here are honest answers to all your questions—plus valuable advice on helping your health the natural way.*

Also by Dr. Alan H. Nittler, M.D.

A NEW BREED OF DOCTOR

Health Questions
and Answers

Alan H. Nittler, M.D.

PYRAMID PUBLICATIONS NEW YORK

HEALTH QUESTIONS AND ANSWERS

A PYRAMID BOOK

Pyramid edition published November 1976

ISBN: 0-515-03723-0

Library of Congress Catalog Card Number: 76-23561

Printed in the United States of America

Pyramid Books are published by Pyramid Publications (Harcourt Brace Jovanovich, Inc.) Its trademarks, consisting of the
word "Pyramid" and the portrayal of a pyramid, are registered
in the United States Patent Office.

PYRAMID PUBLICATIONS
(Harcourt Brace Jovanovich, Inc.)
757 Third Avenue, New York, N.Y. 10017

Contents

Preface

The questions and answers in this book appeared in Dr. Nittler's monthly column in *Let's Live* magazine, 444 North Larchmont Boulevard, Los Angeles, California 90004. They have been reprinted here by permission of *Let's Live*.

Please note: Due to an overcrowded schedule, Dr. Nittler is not able to answer letters or correspond with readers of this book.

Further health information will be found in Dr. Nittler's other book: *A New Breed of Doctor*, sold at health or book stores.

1. Alcoholism

20 Years of Beer-Drinking

Q. *My 60-year-old father began drinking (beer only) about 20 years ago and has made good progress! He quit drinking a month ago (a real miracle), and at that time was consuming between 1 and 1½ gallons per day. Now that he's quit, we want to build him up healthwise, as he's very lethargic, often dizzy, complacent, and so very tired. Will you please recommend a diet that will help?*—M. R., Concord, California.

A. With a history such as this, it is a wonder he is not a walking pathology laboratory. We can say, at least, that there must be liver damage. With this and a poor state of health, anything is likely to happen.

The approach to rebuilding this man's health is twofold. The first is to be sure there is an adequacy of all the basic nutrients. This means all the various minerals, vitamins, enzymes, proteins, fats, and carbohydrates. These must be supplied in abundance and right now! Then there is the specific approach where items with particular values are used. Insofar as liver detoxicants are concerned, there are some on the market which, in my opinion, are good. Beet powder, as packaged in Germany, is also excellent. This is a delightful-tasting preparation which may be sprinkled on your fruit or cereal, or mixed in water for a drink. Various brands of liver powder or concentrate are really valuable. Raw—or desiccated—liver tablets* are a favorite of mine. Naturally, the B complex is essential for the treatment of liver problems. Inositol and choline may be among the most important fractions, but I prefer to use the whole complex in a natural form which includes all the naturally associated synergistic factors. Use a high intake of these.

*See Product Information.

9

I certainly do think that the mono or duo diet is very good for starting the detoxification of the liver. Such menus as grapefruit and celery, grapes, watermelon or carrot juice are types which have proven to be valuable in treating this type of condition. This detoxification diet can be followed for a period of not more than one month. Naturally, the other supplements are to be used simultaneously.

Just as important in the program is *not* to do the wrong things. I believe that smoking can sabotage the program. Coffee is out. Chemicals in the food are out, too.

Incidentally, the use of a coffee enema can be of great value. A strong cup of brewed coffee can be diluted with one pint water and used as a retention enema. This stimulates the liver incredibly. An enema of this type can be used daily if necessary.

Dizzy Spells

Q. My husband gets dizzy spells from time to time. First he gets aggravated, then he has a bitter taste in his mouth, and then he becomes dizzy and loses his memory for a while. When he is having a dizzy spell, he does not even recognize his customers in the laboratory he operates.

His heart is all right, his blood pressure is very good, but his liver is swollen. He has had brain examination, but nothing was found to be wrong.

The doctor has forbidden my husband the use of salt and alcohol, but he will not stay away from alcohol. He drinks three beers or a bottle of wine every day—sometimes more, sometimes less. When he was younger, he drank more, but was never sick then. For a while he stopped drinking altogether, and he had no dizzy spells, and his memory improved.

Since the doctors do not find out what is really wrong, all they give my husband is pills.—Mrs. K. L., New York, N. Y.

A. This is the sort of problem about which it is almost hopeless to try to do anything. You can lead the horse to water, but you cannot make him drink. Your husband is suffering from liver damage, as evidenced by the swollen liver, but he refuses to eliminate the cause—alcohol. Alcohol is not the only cause of a swollen liver, but in this case the two are closely associated and are thus suspect. I would venture that you cannot beat this problem.

As an aside, it would be very important to know what kind of laboratory your husband operates. Chemical exposures are very important in liver disease. Maybe he has an occupational exposure.

Good nutrition demands the proper intake as well as not taking into the system the wrong things. Any deviation from this dual rule can be fatal in such a case as this. Your husband is on "the ropes" and he must act accordingly.

For nutritional help in overcoming alcoholism, read the excellent book *Alcoholism—The Nutritional Approach* by Roger J. Williams, Ph.D., published by the University of Texas, Austin.

2. *Allergies*

Hay Fever and Seasonal Asthma

Q. *I have been suffering from hay fever and seasonal asthma for the last 20 years despite vitamin supplements, with additional Vitamin C, wheat germ and wheat germ oil capsules. Every year I still suffer—four or five months. In order to have some temporary relief, I am obliged to take antihistamines and bronchotabs and use an inhaler when asthma develops. I would like to quit taking these drugs and substitute vinegar and calcium as you have suggested, but I don't know how much vinegar to take daily or what form of calcium to take. About 10 years ago I took cider vinegar and honey, which caused several cavities in my teeth, so I had to stop taking it. Do you agree with this?—G.P., Mtn. View, Calif.*

A. Hay fever and seasonal asthma are allergic diseases. They do respond to Vitamins A, D as well as C and calcium. Calcium should be in the form of raw bone meal. Calcium lactate is useful here but it has other drawbacks. Sometimes calcium metabolism can be enhanced by use of magnesium or silica. Acid is also important and can be taken in the form of apple cider vinegar or hydrochloric acid. The apple cider vinegar and honey mixture you took probably caused cavities, but because of the honey rather than the vinegar. Apple cider vinegar should be taken in water with each meal and sipped like wine: two tablespoonfuls per glassful of water. Also, do not forget the use of pantothenic acid in large doses for allergic diseases. In acute conditions up to 1000 or even 1500 mg several times daily is sometimes very valuable.

Sinus Allergy

Q. For several years I had a bad case of sinus trouble. When I started taking vitamins and minerals, it let up and now I am not bothered with it, but my nose has been sore for several years—so sore at times that I cannot bear to touch it. My doctor said that it was some kind of germ and to use an antiseptic every day. I have done that for about two years and no results. I eat Vitamin C like candy and also take kelp, brewer's yeast, bone meal, Vitamin A, lecithin, Vitamin E, garlic and B complex. Would anything else help?—Mrs. D.L., Otsego, Michigan.

A. Since you are an avid vitamin taker, it will seem odd when I say that you are probably not getting enough Vitamin C. Apparently you are not utilizing it well enough since you are taking a liberal quantity. Also, you should take pantothenic acid. This B vitamin is very valuable in the prevention of allergic states. The dosage can be as high as 1000 to 1500 mg, if necessary, several times daily to control the symptoms. After symptomatic control, you should cut the dosage back to fewer times per day or lesser dosages. If you are still symptomatically controlled, the dosage can be cut even further, and maybe even end up with an intake of 1000 once daily or maybe twice if symptoms develop. (To each his own.) In addition, you should avoid the common allergic foods: milk, wheat, chocolate and sugar. I would guesstimate that 90 percent of all allergic patients would improve remarkably if they were to avoid these foods.

Incidentally, in your multitude of vitamins being taken, you do not mention Vitamin D. This is very important in allergic individuals.

Nasal Allergy

Q. I started having trouble, about five years ago, with my left nostril closing up once or twice a day. I finally went to a nose-and-eye doctor. He gave me some pills that helped some, but he said the only cure was an operation—so I never went back. I have to carry a nasal spray with me and have one by my bed to use at least once a night. It seems that maybe what I need is a good detoxification diet. If this is so, where can I get one? I'm a male, 51.—G.H., Nixa, Missouri.

A. It sounds like you suffer from some sort of allergic reaction. Dr. Carl Reich, M.D., of Canada, has done remarkably well in the field of the nutritional approach to the treatment of allergic reactions. Stress causes alarm, adaption and, finally, exhaustion (Selye's theory). Muscle exhaustion is followed by spasms of the bronchial muscles and tends to cause the restriction of air flow out of the lung. To make a long story short, this results in asthma. The job is to relieve the spasms.

Spasm may be relieved by calcium, but calcium needs Vitamin D. Since most of us don't get enough sunlight in the first place, and seldom get enough outdoor sunlight because it is filtered through the smog-filled atmosphere, Dr. Reich offers large dosages of Vitamin D in his therapy. I suggest you get large doses of Vitamin D for this condition. Of course, you should always include Vitamin A and the calcium with all the other minerals, especially magnesium.

Nasal Allergy

Q. *I have an 11-year-old daughter who chews her nails to the quick and has a touch of sinus. Her nose is often stuffy, and she also has headaches quite often. (The doctor said she had a touch of sinus.) She is very allergic to feathers and will cough all night if she is around them. She has non-allergic pillows. Adelle Davis said the Vitamin C will break up allergy, but so far it hasn't helped, unless it takes several years to break it up. I am giving her multiple vitamins, B complex, Vitamin E and Vitamin C. The allergy to feathers is no problem as long as she is kept away from them. but the nail-chewing and sinus are really big problems.*—Mrs. J. K., Elizabeth, Pennsylvania.

A. Allergies are very complex. There are two simple things to be corrected in allergic patients. First, the administration of acid in the form of betaine, hydrochloride or glutamic hydrochloride, or vinegar, are all important.

This is to ensure proper and adequate digestion. The second thing is to add or correct the calcium balance. Since calcium is only absorbed in the presence of acid, calcium plus acid may help.

Also, recently I have found that five drops of castor oil in water or juice first thing in the morning can help keep nasal passages clear from allergic reactions.

Nasal Swelling

Q. *The inside of my daughter's nose swells up, causing headaches and making it impossible for her to sleep. She went to a specialist, and he gave her some drops, but they do not help much since she can only use them once a day. Can you help?*—G. M., Paramus, New Jersey.

A. Since this condition occurs mostly at night, I would suspect something in the daughter's room is causing her allergic reaction. The pillow is a good place to start. It could be that she is allergic to the dust in the room if there were too many "dust catchers" in the room. Maybe there is a connection with the type of face cream being used, or the toothpaste, or whatever is used on the hair at night. There are many possible allergens to be found in the bedroom.

Nutritionally, high doses of Vitamin C can be of assistance. A liver hormone, yakriton* is a good natural antihistamine. Vitamin A in large dosages is good. Anything that will stimulate the liver is very valuable in the overall treatment.

Hypoglycemia could be an intermediary cause to be investigated here. A drop in the blood sugar level some hours after eating could show up as an allergic reaction. There is only one way to be sure of the diagnosis, and that is to have a five-hour, seven-specimen glucose tolerance test. Proper interpretation of the curve is needed to give the clue to definitive diagnosis and lead to positive therapy.

*See Product Information.

Chronic Nasal Discharge

Q. *Though fairly healthy throughout most of my life, I did suffer from a chronic nasal discharge since early in my teens. Though not painful, the discharge was heavy enough to require almost constant use of a handkerchief. In searching for a cure, I tried the usual treatments—including antibiotics, antihistamines, sniffing salt water, chiropractics and fenugreek—with no improvement. Then, about three years ago in my mid-40s, I noticed a change in my condition. Hay-feverlike symptoms became apparent which did not yield to home treatment. I consulted several physicians, and the final diagnosis was allergy. A desensitization program was begun, but the symptoms became worse with the appearance of asthma. For two and one-half years I continued this treatment, but found relief from symptoms only when cortisone was used. When the allergist finally sent me to the medical school clinic, they diagnosed it as intrinsic asthma and prescribed daily doses of cortisone as the only treatment. I now take 15 milligrams of Prednisolone each day. The symptoms are pretty well controlled, but I still have no sense of smell and must take broncho-dilators each night. I am able to function on my job, but I hate to think of relying on steroids for the rest of my life. Could you suggest any nutritional program that might help?*—J.R., Yakima, Washington.

A. You have a common and very elusive complaint. There are two things that come to mind here. One is the fact that you probably suffer from hypoglycemia, and the other is that there probably is intestinal intoxication. In both situations you need a good sturdy dietary and adrenocortical support program and also a good intestinal detoxification program.

Your body demonstrates poor stamina now and it will get worse day by day on your present regimen.

Post Nasal Drip

Q. *I have a post nasal drip in my throat, which leaves red streaks on the back of my throat. Also, I get muscle spasms on the right side of my neck. When I push my* *neck to the left to relieve this pressure, I hear the bones crack. I was in an automobile accident and dislocated my shoulder and had to have a pin put in it. I didn't use my arm for a while until the pin was taken out. It grew weak and I couldn't raise the arm, so I had to have treatments at the hospital for a while. I've been going to a chiropractor for two years. He says he is trying to build up my left side, but it takes time. I've been taking vitamins and mineral supplements (complete), plus 9 dolomite tablets daily, 400 units of Vitamin E after each meal and one bone meal tablet after each meal. What do you recommend for my condition?*—An Illinois Reader.

A. There is something in this letter that the readers cannot see. It is the way the letter and words and lines are written; they slant to the left. This is evidence to me that you suffer from low blood sugar. Naturally, I am taking a flyer, but I have seen this thing before and feel that it is a problem. The post nasal discharge is also a sign of hypoglycemia. The neck condition is something that is frequently associated with the hypoglycemia. The shoulder condition could have contributed to the problem, too, because it was a stressful situation. All in all, you suffer from nutritional ailments which can be called "dysnutrition." Actually, hypoglycemia or low blood sugar is nothing but a form of poor nutrition.

In my experience, I find that the use of adrenocortical extract is very essential to the quick and effective recovery from low blood sugar. The adrenal cortical extract, incidentally, is not cortisone or cortisol or any other refined faction of the adrenocortical substance, but is the whole adrenal cortex extract in aqueous form. This can be used with no fear of reactions because it is in the natural and complete form. (The refined and purified fractions cause troubles.) Along with the adrenocortical extract, I use a strong nutritional program. The essence of the program is to detoxify the system first and then to rebuild it. This is done by starting the patient on a basic detoxification program and adding to it the necessary items to cause tissues to react in the areas that show deterioration. It is a program which has been proved to be effective. It takes time to effect desired results, but the minimum period which I use it is for three months. This is the time it takes on the maximum nutritional push before the effort can start to be relaxed. Assuming that the results are desirable, the program is then gradually slowed down. Some must be satisfied to rest in an improved state with continued support. At any rate, it is better than the original disturbed picture.

Hypoglycemia is a very real problem that demands expert management under the best of conditions. Great results can be forthcoming, but you must work for them. (See section on hypoglycemia for further help.)

Vitamin Allergy

Q. *I have the following problems with which I trust you will help me: allergy against all vitamins, collectively and individually; continuous heavy heart beat with many skipped beats; hiatus hernia, for which I have been advised not to have surgery.*—Mrs. F.U., Boca Raton, Fla.

A. In my personal opinion, surgical correction of a hiatus hernia should be undertaken only as a last stand. It is a very complex surgical technique and in most of the cases the benefits do not warrant the effort.

Your supposed allergy to all vitamins is another story, indeed. This I cannot comprehend. There must be something else which has not come to your attention. Your skipped heart beats certainly do indicate a deficit of water-soluble B vitamins. I would certainly reconsider what type of vitamin preparations you are taking. There are big differences, to say the least. Foods are the true vitamins! Are you allergic to all foods? It seems to me that you should educate yourself to the best possible degree as to just what good vitamin preparations are. This is not easy to do but the information can be found by research.

If I were to handle your case, the first thing needed would be to have a complete metabolic survey so that the known deficits could be detected. It is then a matter of course as to how these problems are to be attacked. If you are truly as difficult to manage as you imply, it would take all the skill of an experienced nutritionist to lead you through the corrective period into a state of good health.

It should be done slowly and deliberately, following a set pattern. It can be done, though it may be a slow process.

Neck Pain

Q. *Recently I experienced a strange soreness in the area of the gland in my neck. It was very tender, swollen and so sore on the left side that I could barely turn my head. It lasted for five or six days and spread to the left side of my chin at one point. My doctor examined me, prescribed antihistamines (which had no effect except to make me nauseous) and ran blood tests to check for mononucleosis. He suspected an allergy since the blood tests checked out normally. Yet, he admitted that he really did not know what caused the pain, since the antihistamines didn't relieve it. Do you have any ideas?*—A. W., Santa Rosa, Ca.

A. Just because antihistamines do not work on occasion does not mean that the condition is not allergic. I would suspect that your doctor was correct. However, nutrition may help. Vitamin C is important, also Vitamins A and D, and pantothenic acid in large doses.

Vitamin E Allergy

Q. *My 21-year-old daughter is very ill and incapacitated as a result of taking large doses of Vitamin E (600 units) for a period of time to correct a gland condition (no monthly periods for several years) which doctors could not seem to correct with their medications. This corrected the gland condition, but left her with a Vitamin E storage and sensitivity problem. She cannot eat foods with even the slightest amounts of Vitamin E in them without having a hormonal reaction, high blood pressure reaction, swollen liver, swollen glands, swollen bones and severe water retention.*

She has found that eating several tablespoons a day of refined oil uses up some of the Vitamin E in her system and keeps her blood pressure and other reactions at a slightly lower level—but still unbearable, and she is nonfunctional, both workwise and schoolwise.

We are searching for doctors who have done research with Vitamin E in order that we may contact them about her case.

We have already contacted Dr. Evan Shute of London, Canada, who told us that it is quite possible that she is a person with a low tolerance level for Vitamin E.

A. It is possible that your daughter may be allergic to Vitamin E or to some forms of it. I need to know the brand name of the product used as I think that this could be a vital point. Some people are allergic to wheat products or Vitamin E derived from them.

Assuming that she is allergic, I would do the standard things for allergies: Vitamin C and bioflavonoids in large doses, pantothenic acid (about 750 mg per day in divided doses), liver (ten tablets, three times daily) and brewer's yeast (increased gradually).

There are the basics that I would think of on first glance. I would appreciate knowing what happens as she goes into this program.

Vitamin C Allergy

Q. *I am allergic to Vitamin C and almost all vegetables and fruits that contain Vitamin C. All the health food books I have read tell me to take big dosages of Vitamin C, the very cause of my affliction. I am also very susceptible to colds, which I used to suppress with Vitamin C, which I cannot use now because of the intolerance. What should I do? How can I prevent the deficiencies that will result from not eating any fruit and so many vegetables?* —F.W., Los Angeles, California.

A. You say you are allergic to Vitamin C. I do not think this can be so. You may very well be allergic to many different foods which contain Vitamin C or you may be allergic to the chemicals which many times contaminate the vitamin or foods containing it. But I do not think that you are allergic to all forms of the vitamin itself.

First, you need a complete metabolic analysis. It is necessary to know what and how your body is reacting in the process of living and how it works when subjected to the grueling test called the glucose tolerance test. My guess is that you are suffering from hypoglycemia, known as low blood sugar, and probably even from hypoadrenocorticism.

The late Dr. John W. Tintera put these two conditions together with some excellent results. If you do have hypoglycemia, the treatment is much more than just the diet as was suggested by Dr. Abrahamson in the book *Body, Mind and Sugar*. It is much more than hypocalcemia as implied by some; or more than a deficiency of Vitamin B-6; or a shortage of Vitamin C. All of these are important but are not the only simple cause. Dr. Tintera has come the closest in stating that low blood sugar is the result of the failure of the antistress glands, the adrenal cortical glands.

The real and lasting treatment for hypoglycemia is a *combination of all the known methods*. In my experience, I have found that the use of the diet based upon strictly organic and natural principles; upon food supplementation to the maximum degree; upon the usage of tissue extracts, known also as nucleoproteins, cytotrophic extracts, protomorphogens and possibly including RNA and DNA; upon the use of adrenocortical extract injections. This adrenocortical material is an extract of the whole gland, it is aqueous in nature and contains all 32 hormones normally produced by the adrenocortex glands. One of the hormones is cortisone and the material is rated in cortisone activity. Actually, this product in no way acts like cortisone, which I consider a dangerous drug, because it does act as the whole gland would work. There are no cortisone complications from administration of the substance. It is generally nontoxic.

A planned course of action, using these different modes of treatment, leads to a very satisfactory response so that the individual can, for all intents and purposes, live a normal life if he obeys certain basic rules of good nutrition. Results of this magnitude cannot be obtained in any other manner. The injections alone or in combination with a so-so diet cannot do the job. Diet alone cannot do the job in this day and age, due to pollution. The supplementation program is of the essence. One must have the best.

This brings me to the second possibility. You may be allergic to Vitamin C from either rose hips, or acerola berries, or citrus fruits. How about any and all fruits and vegetables? There is good Vitamin C in potatoes, apples, etc., etc. One preparation I use is derived from mushrooms. As far as I am aware, no patient has ever been allergic to this preparation. Don't toss in the sponge, just keep on trying. Sooner or later you will find some answer. Actually, I feel that a five-hour, seven-specimen glucose tolerance test is a must for you. The next must is to find someone who knows how to read the test. Most doctors do not know, nor do the pathologists who are responsible for the laboratories. Sad, but true. They are more interested in doing a three-hour test which is almost totally invalid in regard to low blood sugar.

For more information see my book *A New Breed of Doctor*, now published by Pyramid Publications in paperback.

Brown Spots

Q. *I have developed some brown spots on face and hands but have much trouble with any type of acid: yogurt, acidophilus, bifidus, vinegar, etc., and most especially HCl which gives me a very bad headache. Is this all due to adrenal underfunction? What to do? Fruit also causes a bad reaction the next day.*—Miss D.N., Honolulu, Hawaii.

A. Anyone who is so allergic has problems! I hardly know where to start in trying to answer such a letter. I do know that a complete metabolic checkup is essential. Many things show up in a routine extensive screening approach to diagnosis.

In such a situation as you present, I would be especially suspicious of the possibility of the adrenal gland being very weak. It is probably not knocked out entirely but it is probably severely stunned most of the time.

You need to be detoxified in the severest degree. The problem would be to find the correct approach. I use the mono or duo diet, meaning that certain predetermined foods, one or two of them, should be consumed eight times daily and nothing else taken except drinking water. My favorite basic groups would include carrot juice, or grapefruit and celery, or banana and avocado, or grapes, or papaya and pineapple. Even a diet of watermelon is very satisfactory. You must understand that this single or duo food diet only is to be consumed for the whole two-week period. It does not mean to jump around to one or the other as the mood strikes you. This diet should be supported by the proper vitamin therapy simultaneously. If worse came to worst, I would consider a fast of pure spring water (if you can get it) and a series of colonic irrigations as a starter. Naturally, this regimen should be under strict supervision at all times.

After being detoxified, one could cautiously and with great wisdom gradually develop a dietary intake compatible with abundant living.

Lecithin

Q. *Two years ago, I began following Adelle Davis' nutritional advice, taking all the vitamins, good food and lecithin she writes about. For a year I had horrible crampy pains and diarrhea. I played detective and finally discovered it was lecithin—the inositol in the lecithin, to be exact. Since the inositol acts like an allergy, is there anything I can take with the lecithin to counteract the pain and diarrhea?—K.M., Havertown, Penn.*

A. It sounds as though you might be allergic to soy beans, the usual source of lecithin. Moreover, large doses of lecithin or other phosphorus products will cause a shortage of calcium. Deficiencies of calcium cause spasms in the intestinal tract.

You should also bear in mind that allergies are simply a manifestation of deficiencies: primarily the B complex. Be sure to take plenty of pantothenic acid when testing this theory.

Furthermore, you could be manifesting a shortage of hydrochloric acid. This acid is necessary for the metabolism of almost everything within the body. Of course, protein is the chief element that demands hydrochloric acid.

Reaction to Dairy Products

Q. *Within 48 hours after I begin to consume any kind of dairy products made from cow's milk (such as cottage cheese, buttermilk, yogurt or kefir grains) my heart will begin to skip beats, although I have no gas on my stomach or bowels and no sensation of fullness nor any depressed feelings. Just the plain milk from the cow also affects me as stated above.*—J.R.J., Dayton, Wash.

A. This appears to be a simple case of allergy. It is a specific allergy to milk and milk products.

The usual medical treatment for this condition is the avoidance of such foods.

Desensitization Injections

Q. *I am an allergic person under the direction of an allergist and am getting the desensitization injections. While this is going on, I seem to have a peculiar problem of aggravation of my symptoms on a 3-month basis. This reaction consists of headaches, tightness in the chest, pain in the eyes and feverishness. Can you tell me why this happens?*—Mrs. G.R., Manchester, Pennsylvania.

A. It is difficult, if not impossible, to give a good answer to this problem. It does seem that the body is able to take only so much of the treatment involved and then must evacuate it from the system. In this case, it is the symptom complex you suggest.

Frankly, in my experience, I have found little benefit from the allergic desensitization programs commonly used. It seems, at best, that only temporary relief is experienced by the patient.

The aim of the nutritional approach would be to rebuild the tissues and glands so that they can function normally. My approach is to attack the problem from three different directions. The first is to be sure that all the basic vitamins, minerals, enzymes are given orally and make sure that they are digested. The first phase is to get the nutrients into the blood. The second phase is to get the nutrients from the blood into the cells where metabolism can proceed. The third phase is to stimulate or challenge the cells to use the available nutrients so that the cells will work more normally.

The individual's basic metabolism must be considered. This is why I so frequently state that this patient needs a complete metabolic evaluation. Without this information, one cannot be specific in his therapeutic approach. Once the basics are known, then the program can be instituted with a certain promise of success.

3. Bladder Problems

Bladder Control

Q. *My problem is that I seep constantly and actually wet my clothing when I run or move suddenly. It is so embarrassing. I am overweight, but have no kidney pain or known disorder.*—Mrs. A.H., Albany, Ga.

A. This seems to me to be a clear-cut case of weak muscles. With age, the sphincter muscles in that area tend to become stretched and weak. Another causative factor is childbirth. The usual orthodox type of therapy is to do what is called a repair of a rectocele and cystocele. This lifts the floor of the pelvic area and holds it in place while you are walking around. This is a very satisfactory method of control if you wish to take the "easy" way.

The natural way is to take exercises. This is not easy because it takes discipline and perseverance. There are two techniques I recommend. The one is to tighten the sphincter muscles in that area as one does when the end of a bowel movement is reached. The other method is an exercise which is good for prostate problems in the male. The technique is to raise the knees as far upwards onto the chest as possible, while lying in bed. The knees are then spread wide apart and the soles of the feet are placed together. In this position, the knees are gradually extended while maximum pressure is applied to the soles of the feet. This is repeated 10 times twice daily. It will not be long before there is some noticeable difference in the control of the urine.

Diuretics

Q. *I am using K.B. 11 from the health food store for a diuretic and find that I am allergic to something in it.*

Could you mention something in the natural line that can be used in its place?—D.R.C., Sacramento, California.

From the strictly natural point of view, I can suggest the use of the juice of cucumbers. The dosage may vary from a glassful once daily to two quarts a day. Naturally, this sort of dosage is for a very limited period of time. I have one patient who followed a protein diet for three months to lose weight. He ate nothing but protein foods of animal source. He lost 50 pounds. About two months into the program, his kidneys shut down. He was barely able to urinate and began to fill up with fluids. He was gaining about five pounds per day. His doctors could not help him and they suggested that he avail himself of the facilities of the large medical centers where he could have the kidney dialysis. He refused. He began to use sauna baths on a daily basis. He was able to stay alive that way and control his fluid retention. He would gain five pounds every day that he would not take his bath. He came to me about two months ago in this state. I started him on a complete program which included a watermelon diet exclusively for two weeks. He gradually has improved so that he was putting out about a quart of urine per day. We then decided to have him start on cucumber juice. This helped to the point where he is now putting out about one and a half quarts of urine per day. With this type of output along with the nutritional rebuilding program, I anticipate that we can get this man back to a reasonably normal level of kidney function within the next few months.

Potassium replacement many times will cause diuresis when diuretics have failed. Potassium gluconate is reputed to do the job. Very large dosages of natural Vitamin C can sometimes also do the job.

Naturally, when one retains fluid in the body, one suspects kidney or heart failure. These organs should be checked and given the proper nutritional support as indicated.

Diuretics are dangerous because they cause disturbed electrolyte balance and a lowering of total blood volume. This is of magnified importance during pregnancy. Diuretics and pregnancy do not mix. Every complication of pregnancy and delivery is overactivated by diuretic therapy.

Squamous Cells

Q. *I had a urinalysis done and under the section on Epithelial Cells, Renal, it says many are squamous. As being just an ordinary person I don't know what that means. What about Vitamin A and squamous cells? It has me kind of worried since I am supposed to have many of those cells. Could you please explain what that means. Is it good or bad?*—O.G., Mtn. View, Ca.

A. Squamous cells are the lining cells of the tissues of the bladder. Having so many simply means that you are shedding faster than you should. There is no evidence, medically speaking, that this is of pathological significance.

Enuresis

Q. *Our son is eight and a half years of age and recently, three weeks ago, he began wetting the bed two and three times a night. However, he has no problem with his bladder during the day. After school was out in June, I measured his intake and output of liquids. Although he had a glass of milk each day for lunch and breakfast he did not urinate until four in the afternoon. His pattern seems to be that as soon as he goes to bed his kidney goes on triple duty so that he is wet in one to two hours. Do you have any suggestions for this problem?*—M.B., Holly, Michigan.

A. Enuresis, or nocturnal bed-wetting, is a fairly common complaint. Usually the child outgrows the condition within a reasonable period of time but there are some adults who continue the pattern. In the orthodox field of medicine, there are a lot of tests given which all lead to the usual diagnosis of "cause undetermined." Treatment advised is usually psychiatric assistance.

The late Dr. Christian Volf used high frequency sound phonograph records by a method in which the patient was vibrated by the tones. A series of treatments like this caused the enuresis to subside. They also caused mute children to speak and many other peculiar reactions. He had some 10,000 case histories from his work in Denmark but was not allowed to practice in this country. His findings are not accepted nor available in this country, unfortunately.

Bed-Wetting

Q. *May I ask a question about bed-wetting? Is there any certain vitamin to take? It seems to be hereditary in my husband's side of the family. It is a boy we're having difficulties with.*—Mrs. O.K., Kennewick, Washington.

A. Bed-wetting is a perennial problem. There is no one answer to the problem, but there may be several possibilities. Medically speaking, the services of a specialist in the genitourinary problems are felt to be a must. Usually this consultation draws a blank. Then there are the services of the psychiatrist. Here the effort is mostly a blank, too. The most effective result is to get you, the parent or child, to learn to live with the problem in the best possible compromise manner.

Nutritionally, there are some possible helps. Vitamin C is necessary for proper health of tissue, especially the skin and mucous membranes. From adequate to large dosages of this vitamin can do wonders, sometimes. Vitamin A is also vital to good function of the skin and mucous membranes. The length of time this problem has existed may demand more than the usual effort with this vitamin. Age and size are also important. However, dosages of A in 100,000 to 200,000 units are in order for a temporary period. Large dosages of the fractionated vitamins, even those of organic origin are sold in health food stores, should be used together with natural products containing all the naturally associated micronutrients. (These are the safety valves which protect against damage from the large dosages mentioned above.)

It is conceivable that mineral imbalances could be a causative factor in bed-wetting. Mineral determinations of the blood are sometimes unreliable because there is no way to determine whether the minerals are on the way in or on the way out of the tissues. The urinary excretion studies are more valuable because they reflect what the body is eliminating but they still fall short of real tissue analysis. A new method, analysis of hair to determine mineral deficiencies, is far easier than a biopsy, and is a reliable test. Knowledge of interrelationships of the various minerals is very important, too.

Actually, simultaneous checks of hair, blood, and urine for minerals gives a better overall view of mineral status in the body.

Kidney and Bladder Infections

Q. *My married daughter and mother of a one-year-old daughter has severe bouts with bladder and kidney infection. It comes within minutes, without warning. Medication is the only thing that seems to give relief for a while, but the condition returns. What do you recommend in the way of foods to keep her body free of this infection?*—F.B., Colfax, Washington.

A. You say that your daughter has recurrent bladder *and* kidney infections. It is unusual for the infection to involve both areas. I suspect that this is simply a bladder infection.

Where there is such a recurrent reaction, I first think of hygienic measures.

Asparagus is a good kidney cleanser. So also is watermelon and cucumber taken as a mono diet. Continue the mono diet for 10 through 14 days. Two tablespoonfuls of apple cider vinegar in a glassful of water with meals can also give relief.

Antibiotic-Induced Infections

Q. *You have mentioned the following solution for treating antibiotic-induced infections: 10 percent gentian violet and five percent acriflavin which you insert into the vaginal vault. I have since consulted a urologist and mentioned the treatment you prescribed and was told that the gentian violet was for women only. My condition is of long standing and the symptoms are a painful irritation, burning sensation and excessive redness—mostly at the ex-*

*terior end of my penis. This condition has been the result
of prolonged use of various antibiotics for various ailments. I would be most appreciative and relieved if you
could tell me the proper treatment or treatments I could
use to rid myself of this very distressing ailment.*—C.B.,
Ashford, West Virginia.

A. Actually, the treatment mentioned—gentian violet
and acriflavin, each 10 percent in saturated glycerine—is
for anyone. True, it is messy, but it can be used on any
area of the skin or mucous membranes. This could be used
on the male genitalia as well as the female. It can be used
intraurethally by using a small cotton swab.

However, if you prefer, you could use Corona ointment,
made for cow's udders. It can be purchased from some
farm supply stores. It is a good ointment and can be used
for most anything, even eye infections.

4. Blood Pressure

Borderline Blood Pressure

Q. *My wife is 64 years old. Her blood pressure is 160 over 100. It has been that way for a year or more. Her doctor doesn't believe in giving drugs until really necessary. He says we have to watch and keep it from going higher, but doesn't tell her anything to do to prevent it.* —L.T.F., Charleston, Illinois.

A. When a doctor tells you to watch and see what happens, he is saying, "I hope it goes away, but if not, it has to get worse before I can tell what is wrong." I agree with him that it is not usually wise to give drugs for a blood pressure of this degree. However, it is on the borderline. Drugs have so many side effects and complications that I agree the lesser of two evils is to watch and hope.

Nutritionally, the whole body must be in harmony with all the integral parts. Sometimes a simple thing like calcium lactate will do the job. Sometimes a tablet of dehydrated extract of buckwheat seed and green leaf does the trick. This tablet also contains inositol.

When these measures fail, and they do because of factors which have gone past the point of no return, I turn to a preparation made from the whole root of rawolfia. This is much less toxic than the refined fractions available so readily. A potassium diuretic may reduce blood pressure on occasion.

I personally feel that the increase in blood pressure is not so bad as the side effects of heavy medication most of the time. When I first started practice back in 1946, a woman came to me suffering from a blood pressure of some 260/180. As a young physician, this startled me. I tried to talk her into different sorts of approaches, but she would have none of them. She went her own way. She was already in her 70s and, I found out, had had high blood pressure of that level for at least 15 years. Not only that, she lived by herself and worked in the garden for another 15 years before passing on. This episode made me begin to think about something more than merely numbers and drugs.

High Blood Pressure

Q. *What can be done for a 41-year-old woman with high blood pressure? She has taken magnesium and potassium which helped for a while, but she is very ill again. The pressure is now affecting her eyes.*—K.L., Oakland, California.

A. One of the most important things to learn about high blood pressure is that there is no pat answer to the problem. There is no set regimen which can be applied to the problem to get anticipated results. High blood pressure can be caused by a myriad of things. Many of them are not obvious without a complete metabolic examination. Even then, there may be, and probably are, hidden causes that are undetected. So the first thing on the agenda is a complete metabolic examination.

There are certain items known to have a specific action against high blood pressure. Such things as rutin plus the bioflavonoids, and the B-complex vitamins are very important in maintaining normal blood pressure. Vitamin E can and does cause high blood pressure reactions sometimes, but oddly enough, its deficiency can also cause the same thing. Likewise, large dosages of the alkaline-ash minerals can cause high blood pressure reactions, while in the same breath one can say that shortages of some of these can cause high blood pressure. You mentioned magnesium and potassium as possible cures of this condition. They can be sometimes, but not all the time.

Do not give up here. Many deficiency diseases respond slowly. The proper item in the proper dosage must be taken over a prolonged period of time in order to accomplish the desired results.

However, just bringing the blood pressure down does not solve the problem. Why was the high blood pressure there in the first place? In my experience, I have found that many people with high blood pressure suffer from hypoglycemia.

What is needed here is a complete metabolic examination, including a five-hour, seven-specimen glucose tolerance test and someone who knows how to interpret such a curve.

High Blood Pressure

Q. *I am 59 years old, and have high blood pressure. I also suffer from a change of fluid in the inner ear, which affects my balance. I cannot take drugs. Can you recommend medication from a natural food store?*—J.E.W., Abilene, Texas.

A. You have given a big order here. The high potassium preparations could cause some diuretic water loss, which could cause the blood pressure to decrease and also the fluid to be absorbed from the ear. The preparation I suggest is an extract from watermelon. Incidentally, a diet of watermelon for a few days might be in order for this condition. You could be surprised that this can do so much and give so much energy.

Antihigh blood pressure substances include garlic. This is one that is only good if the smell is *not* removed from the product! Start on a small dosage and gradually build up to the necessary quantity. For instance, Vitamin E could be the causative factor in your case, but in others it could be the reverse. Vitamins B, C, rutin, bioflavonoids and deficiency of other vitamins could be the cause of hypertension. You need a complete analysis and a substantial nutritional program for cure.

Dizzy Spells

Q. *For three years I have been suffering from spells which cause me to feel as if something is turning over in my stomach, followed by palpitation and near blacking out, although I never go completely out. These spells used to last six hours at times and still last two or more hours.*

Sometimes I go as long as three weeks without a spell; then I may have two in a week.

When they first started I weighed 260 pounds and my blood pressure was 300. I now weigh 205 and my blood pressure is 170 over 108.

I've had a hernia for 34 years, but it has never caused any trouble. I've recently had an electrocardiogram and X-rays of the gall bladder, chest and stomach, but doctors found nothing wrong.

I am using juices and taking vitamins I get at the health food store. I am taking niacin, as a lady whose husband has Ménière's disease said that he took it—and the description of Ménière's disease comes closest to my ailment of anything I have been able to discover so far. Also, I do have poor circulation. I am 64 years old.—Mrs. J.A.A., San Antonio, Tex.

A. It sounds as if you have cardiac arrhythmia. The "turning over" sensation in the stomach could very well be the onset of a series of premature ventricular contractions. I would suspect that the rate is either very slow or very fast. In either case, the amount of blood forced into the circulation is reduced so that there is an insufficiency getting to the brain, and due to the reduced blood flow, there is dizziness or near-fainting symptoms. Your past history of obesity and hypertension tend to confirm this suspicion concerning your condition.

The usual remedy from the orthodox viewpoint would be either to try to stimulate the heart rate or to cause it to diminish, depending on whether the heart is going too fast or too slow. For slowing the heart, digitalis would probably be used by the orthodox; and large, almost toxic, dosages would be needed to do the job. In order to stimulate the heart rate, some sort of sympathetic stimulant would be used. Again, this would be less than satisfactory because the dosage needed to accomplish the increased rate would also cause nervousness.

Using the nutritional approach would establish a total heart regimen which would include Vitamins C, E, B complex, along with extract of heart tissue. A tablet which I consider specific for such a state is one that contains the heart extract and B and C vitamins. This tablet I give in hourly dosages, or even oftener when the situation demands emergency type treatment. The hourly dosage should be continued while the patient is awake for as long as needed, even a month or so. When obvious control is attained, the dosage can be reduced accordingly.

By all means, reduce! Being that fat, and at your age, one can speculate on a statistical basis that you will not be around long to discuss your problems.

Taste Buds

Q. What can you suggest to improve one's taste? I am 70 years of age and am taking medicine for blood pressure and cholesterol. Would these affect my taste and what are the side effects of both these medications?—B.L.P., Campbellton, Quebec.

A. I am not certain, but suspect that any drug capable of correcting blood pressure and cholesterol could also affect the taste bud nerves to the extent that the sense of taste is distorted. In this case, to correct the taste situation, all you probably need to do is to discontinue the drugs. Zinc is said to help a loss of taste also.

Sore Throat

Q. I have been having a lot of trouble for about a year with a hurting and raspy throat. The doctor said that my blood pressure was 260 and this was what was making my throat hurt.—Mrs. E. D., Lancaster, Pennsylvania.

A. High blood pressure can be caused by many different and unrelated conditions. It is conceivable that something in the neck can be triggering the blood pressure reaction. For example, the thyroid gland is located in the neck. An overactive gland can certainly cause hypertension and can be felt in the neck region. There can be throbbing, pulsing, fullness and tightness—all of which could add up to pain in certain people.

Protruding Veins

Q. *I am 39 and have large protruding veins in my hands and arms. I have been taking 600 units of Vitamin E each day and 3 tablespoons of lecithin daily for the past two years. Would Vitamin E cause the blood vessels to enlarge? Would silicone injections into the hands, given by a plastic surgeon, be harmful?*—Mrs. S.M., Ontario, Calif.

A. Dilated veins in the hands indicate either some sort of interference with the free return of the blood to the heart or a congestion of the venous system because of too much inflow of blood into the hands. In the former situation, one should look for some sort of mechanical obstruction of the free flow of blood returning to the heart. This block could be either before the blood reaches the heart or in the heart itself. In the latter case, there may be a failure of the heart to expel the blood in proportion to the inflow, due to poor muscle action or arrhythmia of the heart rate or rhythm. It could be that the heart does not work well because of lung damage. In such situations, one would probably demonstrate other evidences of heart failure also.

This, then, leaves us with the idea that there is something wrong with the local circulation or tissue action. In this case, I would first suspect an abnormal thyroid function, probably due to some sort of mineral imbalance. The thyroid is so closely connected with iodine metabolism that it is very tempting to say that this problem could be the result of iodine mis-metabolism. It is conceivable that Vitamin E could be an active culprit here. If Vitamin E is of value to you, I would not cease taking it. Individual symptoms can sometimes be the result of some very unexpected imbalances.

I would not consider silicone injections under any ordinary conditions! I consider silicone to be nonphysiological, and as such, it can be a source of danger.

Low Blood Pressure

Q. *Please tell me what to do for low blood pressure. I keep passing out and injuring myself. The doctors do not know what to do.*—Mrs. M.E., Fort Bragg, California.

A. It sounds to me as if you are suffering from a failure of the adrenal cortex glands. This is a snap diagnosis because I do not know anything else about you other than the letter which is quoted above. You probably also suffer from hypoglycemia. A complete metabolic examination is a must. One just cannot speculate without answers being anything but guesswork.

In summary, you need a completely balanced diet, containing all the essential nutrients in abundance. Minimal daily requirements are a laugh when it comes to therapeutic efficiency. You must take in much more than the "average" in order to get results. Later, when the body is in better health, the dosages can be reduced. The supplements should contain all the naturally associated factors right along with the essential element itself.

In addition to dietary control, you need to have special stimulation of the adrenal glands. This is done by the extracts of the adrenals which can be used orally. Also, injection of the extract of the whole adrenal gland can be used. The aqueous form can be used intravenously, while the oil form is only used intramuscularly.

Low blood pressure is sometimes due to protein deficiency.

5. Body Odor

Kidney Malfunction

Q. *About two years ago my 63-year-old sister started to complain about a smell in her house. She moved, but soon found the new house starting to smell. I always noticed that around my sister the smell or odor was stronger than other parts of the house. I tried to convince her that I felt it came from her. She said that was impossible. She keeps herself very clean. It's neither her lower nor upper body nor her breath, but her skin. She usually eats good food like dark homemade bread, sweet butter, salad, celery, sunflower seeds, some eggs, sprouted wheat, little meat, no coffee, and no medicine. Her appetite is pretty good but she uses flax seed often for a bowel movement.*—Mrs. E.B., Alliance, Ohio.

A. One point that comes to my mind first is that when the kidneys are not doing their work satisfactorily, the skin begins to take over some of the work. Since there are many chemicals excreted by the kidneys, in kidney disease they begin to come out through the skin and an odor is created. In other words, I suspect kidney failure in your sister's situation.

Again, after establishing a full scale optimal nutritional program one can begin to zero-in on the kidneys. Kidneys need lots of good water for proper function. Check the pH of her drinking water. Maybe she is drinking the equivalent of an Alka-Seltzer every time she drinks a glassful of water. Some public water supplies have a pH as high as 8.5 or even 9. This is much too high for good health. The administration of raw kidney tissue extract* is good to help restore proper function to the kidneys. Of course a complete metabolic analysis could reveal other specific needs, one of which could be the answer.

*See Product Information.

Bacteria

Q. *I am terribly worried about my 26-year-old daughter's problem—her strong body odor. She bathes in the morning and before going to bed, uses strong soaps, but toward the afternoon her body odor becomes strong— even outdoors after a shopping spree. Do you have any suggestions?*—C.D., Glendale, Ca.

A. Body odor can be caused by the rancidity of the oils secreted by the body. It can be increased in amount by nervous states and habit patterns. The oils are made rancid by certain bacteria present in the skin. Vitamin E applied locally tends to prevent the oxidation of these oils since it is an antioxidant. Strong deodorant soaps tend to kill off the bacteria on the skin. Unfortunately, the good as well as bad bacteria are destroyed and the bad ones tend to re-populate first. Thus, the ones that tend to putrefy the oils are repopulated first and the condition tends to get worse and worse all the time.

What to do about it is another problem. Many nutritionists tend to feel that it is necessary to re-establish normal flora in the intestines as well as the skin after the normal has been wiped out. Yogurt and acidophilus and other forms of good bacterial cultures taken orally can be used as a skin conditioner to help remove the source of body odor.

6. Bone and Joint Disturbances

Arthritis

Q. *Two years ago I had an operation on my knees. I had arthritis in my knee cap so badly that I could not walk without getting a catch in my knee. The doctor took X rays and said that an operation would have to be done by removing the knee cap. I was in the hospital two months and then moved to a convalescent home for two months. While I was there they applied hot-pack treatments, and all this time I was in a wheelchair. When the doctor let me go home I still remained in a wheelchair. I went to his office every week and he applied an electric massager to my knees. They seemed to heal all right but it seemed to be a little grating there when I bent my knees. Then the doctor started giving me injections of some kind of fluid into the knee cap. He gave me three and after a month or so my knees got worse. Then I got hold of a booklet telling what cortisone would do for someone with arthritis. My knees gradually got worse so I sent three articles to the doctor about cortisone and I haven't heard from him since. He knew all the time that cortisone was dangerous and what it could do to my knees. Now I am asking you to suggest a treatment that will take the soreness out of my knees. Can you suggest anything?—F.J., Florida.*

A. It is quite difficult to accomplish any great improvement in arthritic joints after the damage has been done. Before there is tissue damage, many things can be done and sometimes to great success. However, after the tissues are destroyed, the story is quite different.

I would suggest an immediate intake of cod liver oil. The dosage should be in the range of about two tablespoonfuls each evening along with an equal amount of fresh orange juice. Fresh orange juice does not come from

41

the dairy in bottles which have the same taste day after day and are filled with sugar. Honest orange juice is the order of the day. The cod liver oil should be the Norwegian type. You may be lucky and begin to get results within a few months.

Diet is another important therapeutic agent here. The diet should be mostly raw fruits, vegetables, nuts and seeds.

Arthritis

Q. *As the result of an injury about 12 years ago, I have degenerative arthritis in my neck. X rays show less cartilage and a build up of spurs growing in toward my spinal cord. An osteopath has prescribed Indocin (Indomethicin) to reduce the inflammation and thus reduce the pain. What damage might this medicine be doing in another department? Is there anything else that might accomplish the same results naturally? Do you know of anything that will prevent calcium deposits or dissolve deposits (or spurs) that are already there? I would like very much to get off of this medicine, but cannot until I find something else that will solve the problem. Can you help me?*—J.S., New Hope, Pennsylvania.

A. Indocin is a potent, nonsteroid drug with anti-inflammatory, antipyretic and analgesic properties. Its mode of action, like that of other anti-inflammatory drugs, is not known. However, its therapeutic action is not due to pituitary-adrenal stimulation.

It is not a simple analgesic. Because of the possibility of adverse effects, some of which may be serious, the drug should not be used casually. Indocin affords relief of symptoms. It does not alter the progressive course of the disease.

Indocin relieves pain, reduces fever, swelling and tenderness.

Then follows a series of side effects which take up a whole page of the Pharmaceutical Directory, 1970.

Is there a natural way? Yes, there is. You need to be examined in a metabolic nutritional way so that all the needs of the body are determined from the history, examination, laboratory work or the functional tests. This is the only real way to determine the needs. However, in general terms, the use of a raw diet may do wonders in relieving the pangs of arthritis. It is also necessary to have an optimal intake of all the basic nutrients which include vitamins, minerals, enzymes, proteins, fats and carbohydrates. All the basic foods are needed in one way or another in the body. All are needed to effect a cure of arthritis because normal function in the whole body is necessary.

Osteoporosis

Q. *Could I possibly have osteoporosis? My legs have hurt for 20 years from the knee to the ankle. My doctor tells me he cannot detect anything. If that's the case, why do my legs hurt three-fourths of the time? What would, or could, you prescribe to build bone marrow? I have begun to take bone meal tablets.*—Mrs. J.N.S., New Smyrna Beach, Florida.

A. Yes, you could have osteoporosis at such an early stage there would be no known method of detection. Naturally the use of bone meal is of the essence, but do you have any conception as to how complex this really is? Here are a few of the interrelated factors which must be taken into account.

First of all, the amount of calcium intake must be adequate. Many make the mistake of thinking that since they are taking the correct kind, that is all that is necessary. Not so; the quantity is also important. Next, there must be the proper balance between the calcium and phosphorus. If one goes up the other comes down and vice versa.

Vitamin D is essential for the absorption of calcium. Just because you live in a sunny area does not mean you are getting enough of this vitamin. Vitamin F makes the ionizable calcium more readily available for utilization. The level of sodium must not be too low (low levels impair the absorption of calcium). Potassium plays a reverse role. Calcium is properly absorbed only in an acid state so the nature of the acid-alkaline balance is rather important.

Calcium intake should be accompanied by approximately 20 percent magnesium intake. If this balance does not exist, you might tend to develop kidney stones. The parathyroid gland is necessary for the control of calcium metabolism. Over- or underactivity of the parathyroid can and does play a necessary role in calcium metabolism. Sex hormones are influential in calcium metabolism. Too much male hormone enhances osteoporosis while the estrogen delays the same. Adrenocortical hormones, in their relationship to other minerals, especially sodium and potassium, certainly indirectly influence calcium metabolism. Protein deficiency also adds to the problem of proper calcium metabolism. These are some of the factors involved in the matter of osteoporosis. You can now get a little insight as to why I cannot give you a clear-cut "yes" or "no" answer.

You should also investigate other causes of leg pain. One of the most common is deficiency of Vitamin E. A simple trial test here should suffice as to whether it is valid in your case or not.

The presence of varicose veins can cause pain in the legs, too. You say you have them, so this could be the cause. This demands a proper attempt to cleanse the liver. Congested liver is the primary cause of varicose veins according to my experience. An all-out job of liver detoxification has cured many varicose veins.

Rheumatoid Arthritis

Q. *I have rheumatoid arthritis and hypoglycemia. Also anemia and an underactive thyroid. I am not crippled yet with the arthritis, but keep getting gradually worse. Have had it for about two or more years but only found out it was the rheumatoid type about eight months ago. I am very sore, but only stiff in knees and hips. (My knees are creaky when going up steps.) I also have quite a bit of pain in my shoulders, arms and hips. Lately my hands are very sore. I take a drug—Tandearil—two tablets daily. I have taken two shots ACTH recently. How dangerous a drug is Tandearil? I am discouraged because I feel the low blood sugar diet keeps me in a toxic state because of frequent high protein meals which are acid forming. I would like to go on a detoxification diet, but do not think I can*

under the circumstances. Is there a way I could do this?
—M.M., Unionville, Missouri.

A. I would say you have a most urgent need for detoxification. You are concerned because of the hypoglycemia getting worse during the detoxification. In my experience, I recommend the high *natural* carbohydrate diet with some protein from animal sources. For instance, when the patient first starts the program, I put them on what I call the mono or duo diet. This means that they can have all the carrot juice, watermelon, grapes and grape juice or grapefruit and celery, but only one of these, for two weeks, eight times daily. Sounds drastic? Yes, but it works. This is because the patient is on the detoxification and not on a manipulated normal diet. By this I mean if the patient were advised to eliminate the sugar and starches from the diet, but to eat all the rest of the "normal" diet and then take grapes, for instance, there would be trouble. If the patient eats nothing but grapes for the two weeks, and eight times daily, there is no problem except for a little hunger. But it works without complications except when patients do not obey my instructions.

I had one patient who was on an exceptionally high protein diet whereby she was drinking one quart of milk into which had been placed a dozen raw eggs, every hour. She thought she would die if she did not get her drink on the hour. Amazingly enough, she was able to go on a grape diet abruptly with minimal amount of discomfort and received great benefit.

To get back to your question, you could go on the detoxification regimen and the sooner the better. However, I do believe that one must be under competent observation during this time and be consuming the appropriate food supplements. To do this without these safeguards is asking for trouble.

Perennially Sore Bones

Q. *I have perennially sore bones at the center of my chest. This has been going on for about a year. Whenever I stretch I feel soreness in this area sometimes more severe than other times. I have been to a doctor, but he could do nothing for it. This could have been caused by some weight lifting that I did at one time, but the pain continues even though I quit lifting weights quite a while ago. Do you have any suggestions?*—M.G., Brooklyn, New York.

A. The weight lifting could be the cause of the problem you mention. I do not think you are talking about a strain or sprain, but maybe a dislocation. The ribs can become dislocated sometimes and cause trouble for a long period of time. I would suggest finding a good osteopath or chiropractor who has "the touch." He should be able to correct your problem in short order.

Brittle Bones

Q. *I am 75. Two years ago I fell in my basement and broke my hip. Then, six months later, I fell again and broke the other one and had to have a complete new hip "installed" with all its "hardware." We have been on a good nutritional program for years, so why should it have happened? The bone surgeon said I had good bones and very little osteoporosis, but my arteries are filling up. Now another doctor says after age 45 or 50, the bones do get brittle and that there is need of hormones (estrogen). Is there any natural hormone I can take?*—F.L., Lincoln, Nebraska.

A. Estrogens certainly do improve the health of the bones and reverse the trend to osteoporosis. Bone can be rebuilt by the administration of estrogen. The estrogen, therefore, does produce other results quite apart from the ovarian stimulation. I would advise you to take some of these hormones to help prevent the deterioration of your bone structure as well as to assist in the healing.

The whole metabolism of calcium is very complex. There is a balance between calcium and sodium. If there is a deficiency of the latter, the former could be deficient, too. There must also be a balance between the calcium and magnesium, for example. There are other balances which are important. The acid-base balance is very vital. If there is too much alkalinity, then the calcium is deposited in the wrong places as it is being withdrawn from the right places. This is why arthritics and those suffering from bursitis have calcium deposited in the wrong areas.

One of the chemical means of correcting this abnormal calcium metabolism is to administer ammonium chloride. This substance reduces the alkalinity by combining with the alkaline-ash mineral excesses to break down into ammonia and thence to carbon dioxide and water. This tends to normalize the calcium metabolism and thus to dissolve some of the abnormal deposits. This is far simpler and better, without the harmful effects of so many drugs used nowadays.

Leg Cramps

Q. *What can you do for leg cramps at night? What can give relief at the very moment they occur?*—G.R., Los Angeles, California.

A. There are two temporary measures you can use for relief, but far more important are measures you should begin during the day to *prevent* these cramps. The temporary measures are: Lying on your back and turning your toes upward toward the ceiling. This often breaks the muscular spasm and stops the cramps. If this fails, get up and stand, or walk for a few minutes, or even massage legs until the cramps subside. If worse comes to worst, you may have to apply hot, wet towels, or even get into a tub of hot water. But this is usually not necessary.

Now to correct the *cause* of the cramps. They are due to a deficiency of the following nutrients, or perhaps a combination of them. You will have to review your diet to see which you lack:

Calcium. If you already take enough calcium, then look to your diet to see if you are assimilating it. If you do not have enough hydrochloric acid, you cannot use the calcium you have. Vitamins D and F (unsaturated fatty acids) are also both necessary for calcium assimilation. Some patients are relieved of leg cramps when they add Vitamin D in some form, such as Vitamin D perles, to their supplements. Others experience permanent relief by adding at least two tablespoons of vegetable oil to their diet (in salads, etc.). Many leg cramps occur among those who are on a fat-free diet, when they should not be. The body needs a certain amount of unsaturated fat for well-being and it does not cause added weight. On the contrary, it often helps weight reduction, as well as other body functions.

If you are eating a high-protein diet, or brewer's yeast or lecithin, you need to add extra calcium. The foods previously mentioned, though very helpful, contain a great deal of phosphorus which, in turn, creates a need for added calcium.

One of the best sources of calcium is an enzymatic extract of raw bone meal.

Vitamin B-6. John M. Ellis, M.D., has found that those who are deficient in this vitamin suffer excruciating "Charlie-horse" type of leg or foot cramps at night. He prescribes 50 mg. of this vitamin daily and the condition leaves. However, the whole B complex should be added to the diet when this single B vitamin is used.

Poor Circulation. In this event, I would try Vitamin E on a daily basis first. In the right dosage, which has to be established by each person experimenting for himself. (See Dr. Wilfrid Shute's book, *Vitamin E for Ailing and Healthy Hearts,* published by Pyramid Publications and available through book or health stores.)

In the case of elderly people, if all else fails, niacin, no more than 50 mg taken now and then, has stimulated poor leg circulation, but I prefer to give all of the other measures a fair chance first. Usually, correcting one or more of these deficiencies does the job.

Intervertebral Disc

Q. *My husband, age 33, has a cervical-disc problem caused by osteoarthritis which causes numbness and pain in the left arm and upward. Do you have any comments or advice to help this problem?*—L.S., Rexton, N.M.

A. The intervertebral-disc problem is a form of malnutrition in the great majority of cases. It is primarily a case of mineral deficiencies. Manganese is the main culprit. However, it is absolutely necessary for you to take all the minerals both gross and trace that are needed for normal homeostasis.

Robert M. Martin, M.D., of Pasadena, Cal., has developed a Gravity Guidance System for exercising while suspended by the feet. It, many times, can solve the disc problem. (Available through Dakel Enterprises, Box 433, Soquel, Cal. 95073.)

Gout; "Sweats"

Q. *My son has gout in his hip and has to constantly take aspirin and cortisone shots in order to relieve the pain. This started after he was given antibiotics for a staph infection. What can he do to effect a cure? He is very much interested in the right kinds of food, but isn't sure where to start.*

My own problem is that I had a hysterectomy 13 years ago and have been taking estrogens almost constantly since then. I am always too warm, and the past few months have been having terrible "sweats" nearly every hour. I am sure it has nothing to do with menopause, as I am 60 years old, and the estrogens have done nothing for me. Two weeks ago I stopped them. I can't adjust to heat and cold. In the winter my thighs and legs are always freezing cold.

When I have the "sweats" my head feels tight and hurts. I do have a history of Addison's disease, but that rarely causes trouble any more.—F.B., Ontario, Calif.

A. In my opinion, gout is a metabolic disease resulting from malfunction of the liver. Your son should have an intensive and complete liver detoxification program. He also needs to have a balanced therapeutic intake of all the natural vitamins and minerals, and he must be sure not to take into his body the wrong things.

Kidney detoxification is of the utmost importance also. Urea is a desensitizer, a buffer salt and an osmotic transfer factor, and it helps to rid the body of the excess purine products.

Foods high in potassium, such as leafy vegetables, raw vegetable juices, potatoes and beans, are protective against gout. Cereals, particularly wheat products, should be eliminated from the diet. Sodium in any form should be avoided. No laxatives or antacids containing sodium or sodium bicarbonate should be used. Cherries in any form are very beneficial. All foods which have been devitalized of Vitamin E should be avoided like the plague.

Sweats which appear to be menopausal but are not, are sometimes due to hyperthyroidism. Here the answer is iodine. I use 50 percent tincture of iodine, one drop daily, for treatment. It takes many months to effect a real change here, but it is good.

Paget's Disease

Q. *What can you tell us about Paget's disease? I understand it involves rapid growth of the bone, consequent destruction, regrowth, etc., resulting in a mosaic effect on the enlarged bones.*

In my grandmother's case, this disease is affecting her hip joints and, more recently, her spine. A nerve being pinched is causing her constant, severe pain. Is there anything you can recommend for this condition?—Mrs. N.F., Glenview, Illinois.

A. Paget's disease is called *osteitis deformans.* It was discovered many years ago by Dr. Paget. It usually involved the bones of the skull, but others as well. It is a very deforming condition. From the orthodox medical approach, there is no cure for this situation. The bones will continue to overgrow and cause many deformities of the skull.

Nutritionally, there are some possibilities. First, there must be a complete metabolic evaluation and the person should be put on a basic nutritious diet and supplementation program. This should represent the whole approach in order to get the entire body balanced biochemically and nutritionally. Next, the basic bone problem should be approached. The first product to consider is bone-tissue extract. This substance tends to normalize the tissue whether it is over- or underactive. This substance is an enzymatic extract of raw bone* which is in reality a protein and phosphorus form.

In order to complete the approach, the administration of a good bone meal is necessary for the calcium and other minerals normally found in bone. There must be an adequacy of Vitamin D, parathyroid hormone, calcium, phosphorus, protein and other elements of normal nutrition. Just how successful this program would be depends upon several variables: age of patient, nature of nutritional imbalances in the body, and how long they have been present, and a host of other factors.

Legge-Perthes

Q. *I babysit for a five-year-old boy who is in the second stages of Legge-Perthes. No nutrition books have even mentioned this disease and I don't know where to turn for the answer. He has the usual American diet with enough milk but not enough trace minerals. How can his mother and I improve his diet so he won't have to use a brace for two or three years or more?*—Mrs. W.D., Great Falls, Montana.

A. Legge-Perthes disease is a condition where there is deterioration of the bony structures in the hip joint. From the orthodox point of view, it is incurable and will proceed to get worse. Ultimately, there will be a permanent crippling in the joint. I do not wholly accept this verdict.

Nutritionally, there are many things to do. First and foremost there must be a complete metabolic survey of the assets of the body as well as the deficits. With this information, there is much to be done. All areas of deficit are attacked and the digestive ability is enhanced to take care of the added need. There should be an abundant intake of raw bone meal combined with the marrow.

When you state that there is an adequacy of milk in the diet, I quiver. The regular homogenized, pasteurized pseudomilk that is sold in America today is a far cry from the real thing. Not only are the enzymes destroyed in the preparation, leaving no life therein, but the minerals—including calcium—are made unavailable for human con-

*See Product Information.

sumption. It may go into the mouth, but it does not get into the tissues where it should go. They say incorrectly that pasteurization is the only way to curb the spread of certain milk-borne diseases.

To be blunt, the pasteurization of milk is being done so that the time-honored methods of cleanliness can be relatively ignored when they become too expensive for maximum profit. Also, the shelf-life of pasteurized milk is much longer than that of raw milk. However, raw milk, when it goes sour, is still a good food whereas pasteurized milk spoils and is no longer a food. Certified raw milk is absolutely safe!

In addition to the raw bone meal with marrow, one should take adequate dosages of Vitamins D, A and C. Proper balance of other minerals is necessary for proper absorption of calcium and magnesium. For instance, if there is a shortage of sodium, there will usually be a defective calcium absorption too.

Perthe-Wilkins Disease

Q. *I have just found out that my eight-year-old niece has Perthe-Wilkins disease. Can you suggest any kind of nutritional diet or supplements to help recovery?*—K.H., Kahuku, Oahu, Ha.

A. Perthe's disease is a disease of the hip joint. It is a disturbance in the metabolism of this particular tissue. From the orthodox medical viewpoint, there is little or nothing short of surgery that will be of assistance.

Nutritionally speaking, there are some basic attempts which should be made before accepting surgery as the only answer. First and foremost, a basic nutritious diet with all the fundamental vitamins and minerals. Then you should stress the ones that are particularly important regarding bone metabolism. The calcium is of first importance as a nutrient. In order to metabolize calcium properly, one must have phosphorus, magnesium, sodium, potassium, Vitamin D and all interrelated factors. When all this is done with the aid of HC1 and pancreatic enzymes then we must sit back and wait. It takes time to correct bone damage. If there is absolute destruction of certain structures, they will not be rebuilt. Thus, there will always be a defect. However, we do not know at any one time when the condition has reached the point of no return. One must always try, and many times is handsomely rewarded.

Cortisone and Bursitis

Q. *I have bursitis. My doctor says that all he can do is to inject cortisone. I am very concerned about what cortisone does to some people. Is there any other solution?*

A. Yes. Bursitis can be the result of an imbalance in the acid-base balance of the system. When the system becomes too acid or alkaline, there is a tendency for the deposit of calcium in abnormal places. The bursa is one of the favorite places for the deposit of the abnormal calcium, and eventually, the bursa becomes calcified. Sometimes it causes such acute pain that it is practically impossible to move the limb without crying. It is true that the usual remedy for this condition is to inject the bursa with cortisone. Sometimes, if one is lucky, it only takes one injection. Other times it takes many. But even this does not cure the condition. There is very likely to be a recurrence in the next year or so. Physiotherapy is also of little use.

Nutritionally there is a very simple answer. It is to use a preparation containing 1.5 grains of ammonium chloride, 1.5 grains of calcium chloride, 1.5 grains of glutamic acid hydrochloride, 1.4 grains of calcium phytate, and 0.8 grains of magnesium glycerophosphate.* The dosage to be used is two tablets, four times daily, for about a month and then one tablet, three times daily, for another month. During this time there will be a gradual dissolution of the calcified bursa. Remember the decalcification which takes place here is not a smooth process. The surface of the bursa becomes roughened and very tender. It can be extremely sore, as in an acute spell. To control this pain one can take a capsule containing prostate phosphatase with tillandsia extract.* Two of these capsules, four times daily, should be enough to make the pain more bearable until relief is experienced.

*See Product Information.

There are various medical reports in which Vitamin C complex (bioflavonoids) have been used for bursitis with great success. In some cases 200 mg of bioflavonoids were used three times daily, making a total of 600 per day. In one instance, for example, except for a slight tenderness, swelling and pain almost completely subsided within 72 hours. In another case, 100 mg of bioflavonoids plus 100 mg of ascorbic acid taken every waking hour for three or four days gradually eliminated the pain entirely by the fourth day.

While nutritional treatment is being used, ice cubes in an ice bag or plastic refrigerator bag and wrapped in a towel can be applied for short intervals during the day to help lessen the pain.

Cracking Joints

Q. *I have a friend who has a problem of cracking bones. Every time she moves, her arms crack. Even when she breathes, her back cracks. Could you give any suggestions as to the cause of this condition?*—O.A., L'Anse, Michigan.

A. A very simplified answer to the cracking of the joints is to say that "they need oil." This is not exactly true, but they do get better with the administration of cod liver oil. This is best taken at bedtime with a little orange juice. Two tablespoons of each at bedtime is a good average dose.

Whiplash and Fatigue

Q. *Two years ago I received a spinal injury consisting of nerve-muscle damage (whiplash) and I cannot seem to get on top of same, along with constant fatigue.*

I would appreciate knowing if there is any nutritional treatment that can aid my recovery. I have exhausted the medical profession for care and ventured into the chiropractic profession—whose services I have received for some time now and in whom I have confidence and trust, as they have brought me a long way, considering the type of injury.

I would appreciate any suggestions you can make, as I feel that you will render an unbiased opinion where chiropractic is concerned.—Mrs. F.B.C., Rensselaer, Ind.

A. There are two main features to be concerned about with regard to whiplash. The first is that of the immediate and prolonged effect of the injury and the pressure or tension on the nerves. The second is the stress factor.

In the first situation, it is quite important to avail yourself of the benefits of chiropractic treatments. It seems to me that this is a much better approach to the problem than the usual orthodox methods of rest, immobilization, drug therapy, etc. The manipulative procedures give definite relief to the tension factors and do ultimately give some very permanent help on the long road to healing.

The stress factor is one which is easily ignored. By this I mean the stress on the adrenal glands. Again this takes form in two manners. The first is the stress on the parasympathetic nerves which enervate the adrenals. Exhaustion of these nerves results in dysfunction of the adrenals. The other is the stress on the organism as a whole. Emotional and physical stress combine here to cause an exhaustion of the adrenal cortices. As a result of this exhaustion, the adrenal cortices do not produce enough of the anti-insulin factors in order to properly balance the effects of the insulin produced by the pancreas. In this situation, we then have an excess of insulin with the resultant hypoglycemia, or low blood sugar. This is one of the very definite causative factors in the production of hypoglycemia.

In your situation, I would definitely explore the possibility of this being the cause of your fatigue. The simplest basic test to begin to evaluate the situation is to get a five-hour glucose tolerance test. With this information, you then could start an intensive and complete evaluation of your metabolism and could come up with some satisfactory answers.

Back Trouble

Q. *Can you tell me what to eat to build up the cartilage between the vertebrae? What can one do in a long-stand-*

ing case where subluxation occurs again and again? Mine is of 30 years' standing. I have tried every kind of chiropractor and osteopath. I also tried fasting, but as soon as I resumed eating, the trouble returned.

I decided to space treatments farther apart, and sometimes I go as long as three months. Then I am lame with sacroiliac or lumbars out, and my cervicals causing both physical pressures and mental miseries. I am 67 years of age and still quite active.

I try to live vegetarian, but use some milk and yogurt, an occasional egg or two, and take brewer's yeast. I prefer fruits, fresh and raw. My teeth are not good, so I blend or juice vegetables. Apparently my liver and gall bladder are weak points, for I don't tolerate much fats or oils or nuts.

I have tried to exercise moderately. I walk a good deal when my back is up to it. Exercises seem to get it out, however, so then I rest and begin again.

Can you suggest anything, nutritionally or otherwise, that might help?—E.M.C., Arlington, Va.

A. You have problems! Even though this is a severe problem for you, it is a very common picture of people in general. There is nothing like a backache to stimulate a conversation at a party. Just mention how you are doing and there are several who can come up with stories which sound a lot worse than yours. But the fact that backache is such a common thing does not make it right. The big problem is why so many people are affected with this condition.

Disease is caused in certain circumstances by various factors, such as age, sex, occupation, place of residence, heredity, past history, and nutritional factors. You can do something about your nutritional status at each and every meal, beginning right now. What is accomplished is often way beyond expectation. One never knows until he tries.

Your problem demands a complete checkup from all angles: historical, physical, clinical, functional and even "laboratorical" (if you allow me to coin a word). Let the findings speak for themselves. Where weaknesses occur, do not let prejudice interfere with common sense and a corrective program.

Of course, chiropractic treatments are helpful. They correct the subluxation or dislocation of the various bones and joints. But, unless something is done to correct the nutritional health of the individual tissue, there will be a recurrence of the condition. The corrective manipulations are only temporary unless definite nutritional measures are taken at the same time. In your situation, I presume that mineral balance is of the utmost importance. All the minerals in proper balance are essential. Maybe the one of most importance is manganese. Manganese, in proper balance, strengthens the ligament tissues. It is the weakness of the ligaments which allows the subluxation to recur.

You also include information which sounds as if you probably suffer from protein shortage. Maybe this is primarily due to the inability to digest protein, which is a very common reason for people to become vegetarians. Since they cannot digest protein properly, they feel better when they do not eat it. You must do all within your power to stimulate your digestive apparatus. One of the most important needs in insufficient digestion is to provide and get into the system the very things which the individual has difficulty in digesting. Hydrochloric acid is an important aid in accomplishing this end.

This problem is discussed helpfully in Linda Clark's book *Secrets of Health and Beauty*.

Back Trouble

Q. *I had a back operation as a result of an accident. One of my discs was taken out. Although the pain disappeared, I always had a kind of weakness in the lower spine where I was operated on. I felt comparatively good until the condition worsened gradually and steadily until I have pain most of the time—not in the spine, but the sciatic nerve in both legs up to the pelvis. I live on excellent organically grown food from my garden: green leafy vegetables, nuts, grains, and seeds. I am otherwise in fine mental and physical health.*—Mrs. L.H., Clear Lake Park, California.

A. At this point you are in great need of all the basic nutrients including protein. You claim to have them in your diet, but I doubt that you can consume enough of them that way. It is almost a *must* to take the various ones in tablet form. In addition, I would consider exercising while suspended by your feet. There is an expensive "antigravity apparatus"* which allows you to hang by your feet, head down. In this position, there is none of the usual pressure on the discs and nerves. Pain is relieved as, exercising in this position, the vertebrae tend to spread apart. Dr. Martin says there is absolutely no reason for back surgery when this sort of exercising is combined with diathermy and other exercises.

Coccyxdenia

Q. *My doctor has just confirmed through X rays that I have coccyxdenia and that, as best I can remember, sometime approximately 23 years ago I fractured my coccyx and tore some ligaments (I am now 30 years old). Although my lower back has always been extremely sensitive to the touch, it wasn't until about three weeks ago that I began having minor pain when sitting or lying in certain positions. My doctor feels surgery for removal of the coccyx is in order, but I would like to avoid surgery on such a crucial area as the spine, if possible.*

I would like to know if there is some nutritional therapy I might use that would correct this without surgery and if trouble such as this can sometimes be a source of minor emotional disturbances since the spine ties in with our central nervous system?

I would also like to know what measures to take in order to prepare myself for surgery if it is necessary and what nutritional measures to use for the speediest healing process without scar tissue possibilities.

Does this condition ever correct itself and would surgery such as this affect the flexibility of the spine in the future and prohibit exercises that involve the spine such as yoga, which I enjoy doing?—Mrs. D.S., Scottsdale, Ariz.

A. The only answer to nonunion of fractured coccyx bones is surgical removal. There is no way to make a small piece of bone stay in one place long enough to form a callus necessary for healing bone fractures. You are talking about the tip of the tail bone, and it is not a vital area

*See Product Information.

as you seem to think. It is nothing like the area of the back farther up where the spinal nerves are located.

I know of no nutritional measures for healing such a situation.

What to do to prepare for surgery is another story. You need an abundance of Vitamins A, D, C and B complex. Of course all vitamins are needed when the body is subjected to stress . . . needed in more abundant doses than under normal living situations. You also need an adequacy of protein. Zinc is another element which enhances healing. A total nutritional picture is needed not only for normal living but also for times of stress.

Ligament Trouble

Q. *What causes trouble with the ligaments? Can any special foods or diets help in their repair? I have trouble in the lower-left back which was diagnosed as ligament trouble by a neurosurgeon, orthopedic surgeon and others, but their only recommendation is a back brace.*

Exercises increase the pain, although walking and jogging help me to keep feeling fit.—Mrs. M.C.K., Los Alamos, N. Mex.

A. Ligaments, like any other part of the body, are nourished by the foodstuffs found in the blood. Obviously, the ligaments do not require the same sort of diet as is needed by the heart or the brain. This can easily be proven in the laboratory.

If you are having problems with the ligaments, I would first look at the blood supply to the tissues themselves. If this is found to be in good order, my next point of search would be to investigate the quality of blood delivered to the ligaments. This would involve the mineral content primarily. (I say this with tongue in cheek because I am assuming that your diet contains all the vitamins and proteins and fatty substances in proper balance. However, the minerals are the critical point of investigation.) We know that *all* the minerals, or electrolytes, should be in adequate amount, but manganese* is the one of great importance to the ligaments.

*See Product Information.

In such a problem as you present here, there may be osteoporosis, or weakening of the bone. Control of this situation demands adequate calcium and phosphorus intake and/or raw bone meal* along with hormonal stimulation, such as ovarian stimulation in the female and testicular stimulation in the male.

Staph Infection of Bone

Q. *My husband had a hip operation about three years ago and ended up with a terrific "staph" infection—the worst kind, the doctors said. This infection gathers and breaks on the average of 6 to 8 weeks and then drains for a week or so. We are getting so worn out with it and would appreciate it so very much if you could help us. In reading about autotherapy, we feel that that is the answer.*—Mrs. C.A.D., Bayfield, Colorado.

A. I gather you are asking about treatment for a staphylococcal infection of the joint or bone. It sounds like osteomyelitis. The first rule of thumb concerning such a chronic condition is to be sure that the body is in proper balance with all the nutrients. This is not accomplished by taking the best vitamins available. When a problem exists, it is necessary to have the body analyzed. This means a complete metabolic checkup and analysis. When the facts are available, then your specific deficiencies or imbalances can be ascertained. It is only logical to follow such a program because one must have the wherewithal to build antibodies and other forms of weapons against the invading staphylococcal forces.

You mention autotherapy. This is a very simple natural method of curing diseases. It is practiced every day by animals when given a chance by their oversolicitous and overzealous owners and veterinarians. Dogs and cats simply lick their wounds which are exuding a pus discharge. This discharge contains all the organisms present in the wound, and taken internally cause the immunological functions of the body to get into action and build antibodies necessary for the job at hand. This sounds horrible

*See Product Information.

in this day and age of sterilization and cleanliness. Practically, it is good. Have you never had an infected scratch on your hand to which you applied this method with good results? I have many times. Healing sometimes comes so quickly that I hardly realize what has happened. A dog does something else, too. His tongue cleanses the wound. If the wound is below the surface, he licks and licks until it drains out. When it drains, his body then responds in the immunological manner needed to throw off the infection. Staphylococcal infections such as this should respond rather quickly to this method.

7. Chiropractic Adjustments

Q. *Please tell us if treatment by chiropractors and physical therapists is harmful to arthritis and rheumatism.* —E.P., Pekin, North Dakota.

A. Chiropractic and physiotherapeutic treatments are not necessarily harmful in the treatment of arthritis. It depends upon the type of arthritis being treated. For instance, if the bones are osteoporotic, it would be unwise to manipulate. However, there are many times where a loosening and manipulative treatment would be of great advantage to the patient. In my practice, I always welcome the cooperation of a good chiropractor.

8. Cholesterol and Artery Conditions

Hardened Arteries

Q. *What procedures and/or treatment can be procured to help alleviate and/or cure the following conditions?*

1. *Hardening of the arteries*
2. *An atonic bladder—large and distended—which does not empty completely, leaving residual urine, causing infections, etc.*

—J.B., N. Miami Beach, Florida.

A. Hardened arteries are commonplace in the USA today. We have been conditioned to blame cholesterol for this. Actually, cholesterol is necessary for the production of adrenocortical hormones, sex hormones and bile salts. If we do not have enough cholesterol, we suffer from an underproduction of these vital substances. I believe high triglycerides (fatty substances) are more likely to be involved.

In my experience I find that high triglyceride levels, a contributing factor, can be brought under control by dietary corrections. If we are eating enough natural fat, then hardened arteries do not occur. These natural forms include the saturated, unsaturated and polyunsaturated fatty acids, not the man-made fats, which are the hydrogenated or solid fats such as margarines and solid cooking fats.

I am also convinced that high triglycerides are the result of high carbohydrate intake in man-made foods like white sugar, white flour and white rice, instead of honey, natural whole grains, fruits and vegetables. Hardened arteries can affect various parts of the body since the blood vessels reach all parts of the body. This is also why patients can have many different and apparently unrelated symptoms. Deficient blood supply causes malfunction wherever it happens and it happens when there is hardened arteries.

Treating an atonic bladder is an entirely different story. It is a matter of getting a complete nutritional program including specific therapy for muscle action. Some patients have been helped. Protein, manganese and magnesium chloride can strengthen atonic bladder muscles. There is a 10:1 neuromuscular concentrate of wheat germ oil* which could be of value here.

Atherosclerosis

Q. *My memory is poor but I believe I have read that lecithin is a remedy indicated for atherosclerosis, which I have. During the last several years I have taken orally, literally, gallons of lecithin but it seems none hit my blood stream or if it did it was altered in my body on its way there. I have never noted any effect therefrom. Is it probable or even possible pure lecithin taken "intravenously" would be an effective and harmless therapy for atherosclerosis?*—A.C.

A. Lecithin should never be taken intravenously. It would cause clogging of the smaller arterioles and this would result in death. Lecithin is reputed to help dissolve atherosclerosis. For those who take it orally, it may be possible that absorption is not complete in some cases.

There are other ways to attack the atherosclerotic problem, however. For instance, magnesium orotate* is reputed to help dissolve the hardened fractions of the arteries. Polyunsaturated fatty acids do help to reduce cholesterol and triglyceride concentrations in the blood and thus help alleviate the hardened arteries.

Cholesterol

Q. *I have been given to understand that Vitamin E, lecithin, pectin, and vanadium (Scientific American, July 1972, pg. 59) are all anticholesterol agents. What precisely do they do and how does one determine how much to take? Could a specific dose of say, vanadium compensate for several pieces of cake, etc.?*—E.H. Hartford, Conn.

*See Product Information.

A. I have no information concerning vanadium. Cholesterol is a substance which has been the "fall guy" for many a year now. It is well known that cholesterol is mainly manufactured within the body and that the amount taken in the diet is only a minor percentage as represented in the blood. Cholesterol is necessary for the manufacture of certain sex hormones as well as those produced by the adrenal cortex. Deficiencies of cholesterol cause problems in these areas.

Triglycerides (fatty substances) are almost always associated with an elevated cholesterol and are really the elements which should be condemned for causing hardened arteries. These triglycerides come mostly from the ingestion of processed man-made carbohydrates and man-made fats and oils. These are the dangerous foods. Lecithin is a fat soluble element which tends to neutralize triglycerides and other harmful lipids so as to emulsify and eliminate them from the body.

Vitamin E is more of an antioxidant. This means that fats are prevented from becoming rancid if enough Vitamin E is present. This is not really an anticholesterol factor but may tend to guard against hardening of arteries.

I thoroughly condemn the concept that if one takes enough of the preventive substance, he can indulge in the bad item (cake in your case) whenever he wishes. Sooner or later there will be the price to pay.

The best way to reduce the cholesterol in your system is to go on a raw diet. Your body needs the saturated fats as well as the unsaturated and polyunsaturated ones. Too much of any of these is not right either. Eat a balanced meal at all times. The highly processed carbohydrates (those manufactured by man) are the culprits, along with the man-made fats such as oleomargarine, shortenings, etc. Anything that is homogenized is suspect.

Value of Lecithin

Q. *Much is written about the value of lecithin in the diet. What is the exact function of lecithin? Can an overdose be harmful?*—S.T., Jackson Heights, New York.

A. Lecithin is a phospholipid, meaning that it is a fatty

substance which contains phosphorus. It is a fat solvent, meaning that it dissolves fat. This makes it valuable in attempting to remove fatty deposits from the tissues, and cholesterol from hardened arteries. Since phospholipids constitute upwards to 20 percent of the nervous tissue, it seems logical to strengthen the nerve tissue when a cold is threatened. When you are in the early phases of a cold, large doses of liquid lecithin, say two tablespoonfuls for four doses, spaced throughout one day, should help the cold to vanish.

Overdoses of lecithin are the equivalent of calcium deficiency symptoms since too much phosphorus is anticalcium.

Obliterative Arteriosclerosis

Q. *The large aorta associated with the mesentry gland is constricted to the extent that I am unable to eat normal amounts of food. Because of this, I am now 25 pounds underweight. I do not gain weight on my limited food intake. Doctors say this condition can be corrected by surgery, but I am not yet willing to undergo it. Normally, the discomfort is not too bad, but occasionally the pains and discomfort are quite severe. I am 50 years old and in my younger days was quite active as a ballet dancer. Are there some natural ways of dealing with this problem? Are there some food supplements you would particularly recommend for this condition?*—J.B., Teaneck, New Jersey.

A. It sounds as if you are talking about obliterative arteriosclerosis of the abdominal aorta with involvement of the mesenteric arteries as well. The actual site of this problem is of more interest to the surgeon than it is to us. There are several things to be done in the immediate future. First, and maybe foremost, is the use of Vitamin E. The starting dosage would be a matter of guessing. A low amount to begin with probably would not cause the blood pressure to rise, etc. I would then, if the situation warranted, increase the dosage slowly to maybe double that amount. I prefer use of several different products, rather than excessively large doses of only one type.

Other items of great need would be Vitamins C, B-15, B

complex and all the other basics. The use of lecithin, inositol, choline and methionine can be of great assistance.

All of these must be put into the system. However, the body can only utilize a certain amount, so you are limited by the capacity of the body to respond. The body can be over-pushed, so this must be handled with wisdom. Each patient is unique.

9. Circulation Problems

Circulation

Q. *We eat no processed foods, make our own Swiss cereal, take lots of vitamins and do all the things we know to live healthfully, yet I have trouble with my legs. I get a burning feeling in the legs, not only when I am off my feet, but when I'm on them. Now I can see the veins breaking where I feel the pains. Can you help me?*—D.G., Pittsburgh, Pennsylvania.

A. Nutritionally there are a few things that occur to me. The use of B-3 (niacin) and B-6 can do things for the circulation and relieve the tingling to a great extent. Naturally this and other vitamin suggestions imply the usage of the natural and organic preparations. I really prefer the low potency products as a starter and then move into the higher potencies if the need still exists. Vitamin E is also important here. The dosage is quite variable and may be quite large depending upon your individual needs. Start low and gradually increase as the situation demands. Vitamin B-15 is also in this category but is not available in the United States as yet. (Incidentally, if you people want to have the advantage of vitamins which are not available to you over the counter, it is your duty to put pressure on the authorities so that they will make them available, at least under the doctor's supervision.) There is also the need for calcium which, when deficient, could cause the same sort of symptom complex as you describe.

Finally, last but not least, the need for hydrochloric acid in the stomach is absolute. Without it many nutrients cannot be absorbed.

Cold Hands and Feet; Nausea

Q. *Could you please advise me as to the cause and remedy for my problems? My hands and feet are always cold (especially my feet). My stomach is so sensitive that merely a little odor will cause me to feel sick at my stomach all day. I also have a tired, weak feeling in my knees.*—Mrs. C.W., Everett, Wash.

A. Your problems represent some major deterioration processes going on within your body. You do not have time to waste in getting on a good nutritional program of detoxification and rebuilding of tissue.

The cold hands and feet represent one or both of two conditions. Either the blood supply is interfered with in getting to the limbs or the tissue utilization of oxygen is decreased. I suspect that both factors are important in your case. Two of the main factors to help remedy this condition are Vitamins E and B-15. Both of these items increase the per-minute bloodflow to the limbs. In addition, the oxygen utilization factor is enhanced. Thus the tissues are able to get a higher percentage response to the oxygen than would be expected under the circumstances.

Of course, Vitamin E is available in many places. I firmly believe that the total E complex is most desirable and not just the d-alpha tocopherol. The B-15 is not available in the U. S. at this time. Do not be fooled by names that sound like B-15; these products do not contain enough of the item to be worthwhile.

Another thing that comes to my mind when you talk of such symptom complexes is poor liver function. I do not think a patient can have so many symptoms unless there is some degree of liver damage present. A good liver detoxification program should be instituted at once. In your case, your low threshold of nausea is a clue to liver malfunction. You probably have low blood sugar, too, just to top it off. The sooner the treatment is begun, the better.

Failing Memory

Q. *My 75-year-old brother's memory is failing. His doctor told him to go on a heavy protein diet and also to get injections of B-12. I'd appreciate hearing your opinion and advice.*—M.P., New York, New York.

A. The advice given your brother is good as far as it goes, but there may be something more that can be done. One must be very sure that there is a balanced diet, and there is no intake of chemicals used for preservation, as well as the artificial foods which contain nothing of great value, but are loaded with calories. It is these pseudofoods, in my opinion, that cause many of these problems. They cause many vitamin deficiencies because they rob the body of vitamins in order to detoxify the chemicals. Nor do foodless foods supply the items needed by the body. So deficiencies are two-fold.

Yes, something can be done. Just get busy with the balanced diet and a good therapeutic dosage of the vitamins and minerals needed for basic needs. Lecithin is a good nutrient for brain function, but this must be balanced with calcium because the excess phosphorus in the lecithin could cause a calcium shortage. The usual vitamins, especially the B complex, are necessary for healthy nerve function. Give your brother plenty of good B complex, especially the thiamin group, including niacin and B-6. Vitamin T, derived from sesame seeds, is a great memory improver, too. Vitamin E, ditto.

Vasoconstriction of Arterioles

Q. *I am 47 years old and recently had the flu with a temperature of 102°. Since then I have very cold feet, and if I don't warm them with hot water, areas of my foot, i.e. toes or heel, will turn absolutely white. Do you have any suggestions which might help this condition?*—M.C., Riverside, Cal.

A. It sounds like you are suffering from the vasoconstriction of the arterioles in that area. From your description of the flu, which left you debilitated, I would suggest an evaluation of your thyroid function. It is also possible that you have brought to the surface a preexistent condition of hardened arteries. In this case you should have abundant amounts of Vitamins C and E for sure.

10. Dental Problems

Dental Problems

Q. *I have developed high blood pressure, now being 23
above what has been considered normal for me for the last
few years. My physician has prescribed tranquilizers and
he said the high blood pressure is caused by tension.*

*Today, upon visiting my peridontist for the usual three-
month checkup and cleaning, he found an abscess in
which I had no pain whatever as a symptom. He said it
had caused considerable bone loss. He operated, etc., and
said the tooth wouldn't last much longer due to the root
exposure (due to previous gum operation for pyorrhea). It
is the last molar and loss of same means I simply will not
have a tooth, as it cannot be replaced with a false tooth.
My question, therefore, is, can some sort of food supplement such as extra calcium in the form of dolomite or
bone meal perhaps cause the bone to fill in where it has
been destroyed, or maybe make it stronger to resist further
erosion in the future? What do you suggest regarding the
advisability of extra Vitamin C? The dentist said it was
caused by a small particle of food working its way into the
area between the roots and bacteria causing the abscess. In
other words, I am interested in doing something to help
that area to be more resistant to future attacks. At present
I take brewer's yeast, liquid lecithin, Vitamin A, Vitamin
E, powdered protein and 900 mg of the Vitamin C complex. I also take three grains of thyroid daily, plus estrogen, both of which are prescribed by my physician. For
the greater part I have always been in near to perfect
health and I depend heavily on natural foods and have
done so for over 30 years. I also take about 10 to 12
ounces of fresh vegetable juices daily. Is there anything
I can take to further strengthen my resistance to this*

thing? Please advise me.—Mrs. M.G, Warwick, Rhode Island.

A. First, your high blood pressure could easily be caused by the abscessed tooth. It could already be cured.

In my opinion it is a gross error to do a gingivectomy. This procedure causes more loss of teeth than most anything else. The best thing for gum health is a soft toothbrush. Keep it busy massaging your gums. In a matter of a week or so many gums can be brought back to near normal.

Yes, a good calcium source is necessary to protect and repair teeth. I prefer a raw bone meal and certain organic forms of calcium from plants. As for dolomite, I am not in sympathy. This is a combination of calcium and magnesium carbonate.

From a clinical level, it is my experience that when dolomite is consumed, even if blood and hair content levels are high, symptomatically, the body still needs calcium on a metabolic level.

Vitamin C should always be taken with calcium. Lecithin, which is a phospholipid and contains phosphorus, also causes an extra need for calcium. Not that lecithin is not important but it should be balanced with the use of calcium.

Peridontal Disease

Q. *I am 50 years old and have never had a tooth extracted. I recently went to the dentist and had my teeth cleaned and since my "bite" was not right, I had this done. The dentist said I have cavities which need filling and also the bone in my jaw is receding and he suggested bone graft. He said this was all due to peridontal disease. I am wondering if I could help this situation by taking lots of calcium and bone meal, as I do not like the idea of bone graft. I read in a health magazine that peridontal disease was a nutritional deficiency and so it would seem like the proper vitamins and minerals would correct this.*—Mr. W. J., Ocala, Florida.

A. Peridontal disease is a very prevalent disease today. It is also very popular. It is due to the receding of the bone from the tooth socket so that infection can enter and cause the loss of the teeth. Gums are also involved. It is a deficiency disease and no amount of mechanical correction of the difficulty after it has formed can correct the cause, which is malnutrition. Factors needed in abundant levels are: calcium, magnesium, Vitamin C, B complex factors, Vitamins A and D and all other macro- and micronutrients. The gums are only a small part of the evidence of the degeneration of tissues of the entire body when malnutrition exists.

Malnutrition can and does exist even when a person has enough food to eat. It is the type of food eaten and how it is prepared and digested which are the important factors.

Care of the teeth is also very important. I believe in the use of a very soft-bristled brush made of nylon fibers. (Sorry, this is a point where I've changed my mind since writing on the subject in my book *A New Breed of Doctor*.) The nylon must be soft so that the gum can be brushed vigorously. Scrub your gums and do not worry about the teeth. They will be cleaned in the process. Do not merely wave the toothbrush at the teeth. This never cleaned any tooth. Get in there with a soft bristled brush ... and scrub! Dental floss should be used to clean between the teeth.

Caries

Q. *I am only 26 years old but the dentist has already pulled three of my teeth. There are several cavities to be filled. I was raised on an organic farm where we had raw goat's and cow's milk, plus fresh produce. I did eat commercial candy in spite of disapproval and had fillings in my first teeth. We also took bone meal powder with a low magnesium ratio. For over the last fifteen years, I have been careful to avoid all commercial carbohydrates and used only honey or raw sugar and mostly fresh fruit and dried fruit. Could you give me any suggestions or advice for my difficulties.*—M.R., Zephyrhills, Florida.

A. First, you mention certain vitamin preparations and ask my approval. I cannot give my approval, but can suggest that homogenized bone meal is not the best. Other than that, the products seem to be OK.

From your story, the main and obvious thing is the consumption of sweets. The so-called raw is white sugar with molasses added. Even more serious is the apparent lack of hydrochloric acid in your system. If I had to make a guess as to the cause of your difficulty, I would choose the lack of this acid.

I shudder at the prospect of your losing so many teeth. However, there are dental methods where the teeth can be capped, crowned and all sorts of things done to maintain your bite. This should be done if at all possible.

In the meanwhile, be sure to maintain the hydrochloric acid intake. This not only enhances your intestinal digestion but also the calcium metabolism on a cellular level. This local digestion or metabolism depends very much on the proper circulation of the lymph. If there is "constipation of the lymph" it means that the nutrients do not get to the cells as they should and the waste products of metabolism are not removed as efficiently as possible. These are both very important factors in the overall nutritional picture.

Fluoridated Toothpastes

Q. *I do not understand about toothpastes. Claims are made that fluoridated products are best, but then some nonfluoridated products are claimed to be even better. What is your opinion about the use of toothpastes?*

A. As we know, the mouth contains teeth to be used for mastication of food. This is a very essential function, and while it is in progress, the food is also mixed with saliva which biochemically and enzymatically aids in the breakdown of foods.

The aftereffect on the teeth will vary as to what kind of food was eaten and how long it was masticated. Some foods, like apples, cleanse the teeth. Here the abrasiveness of the apple pulp and juiciness of the fruit cleanse the teeth of residual particles. The particles are gone but some juice residue remains on the teeth for a while until it is rinsed off by the saliva. Some foods are sticky and tend to cling to the teeth. Such foods usually include the highly processed carbohydrates like cake, cookies, bread, etc. It takes a long time for the salivary flow to cleanse the teeth after these foods are eaten.

Certain bacteria normally live in the oral cavity. When we use chemicalized toothpaste, we change the bacterial flora in the mouth. Halitosis, in at least one instance, is caused by disturbed bacterial flora in the mouth. What is usually recommended is more chemicals in the toothpaste, gargle or mouth wash to make the situation even more abnormal. Whenever we sterilize the mouth, all the bacteria are eradicated but the "bad" organisms are the first to repopulate the area so more sterilizing becomes necessary.

It is my opinion that the use of chemicalized toothpaste, gargles and mouth washes causes a disturbance of the normal bacterial flora in the mouth. I recommend the use of "elbow grease" on the other end of a soft-bristled toothbrush. Get in there and scrub those adhering particles from between the teeth. No toothpaste is needed. If you, as a creature of habit, need to taste something different, you can use sea salt available in health food stores. But this is not necessary for good cleansing. Dental floss is to be used between the teeth.

It is not the fluoride in the toothpaste or water that cuts down on cavities, but the calcium, phosphorus, magnesium, et al., present in the diet. It is also important not to eat "sticky foods," not only because they stick to the teeth and cause abnormal bacterial growth, but also because they, almost universally, do not contain the above-mentioned essential elements.

Fluoridation of water supplies is quite a hoax. It only delays cavity formation, does not prevent. It works only on teeth in formation stage, so application via toothpaste is useless. It neutralizes magnesium which is involved in about 70 percent of all enzyme reactions in the body. Since enzymes are living substances we should preserve them, not kill them with fluoride. Incidentally, the Water Pik is not healthful. The pressure of the water under the gums forces bacteria into the blood stream. This is not desirable.

Erosion of the Teeth

Q. *Please advise me what causes erosion of the teeth. What measure can be taken to halt this condition once it has started? My teeth are in excellent condition, but I seem to be in the beginning stages of this condition. My health is excellent also.*—S.T., Jackson Heights, New York.

A. The first thing I think of is that you are consuming something which is causing the erosion. One thing that many people do is to suck on Vitamin C tablets. This acid can and does sometimes cause an erosion of the enamel. Another thing that can cause this is blackstrap molasses. If either of these items is used, and they should be for your health's sake, you should brush your teeth after taking them. The same applies to drinking lemon juice in water. I have heard that oranges and grapefruit will cause this same erosion, but I am sure that this is only when one consumes an extensive amount of the citrus. I would certainly suggest continuing these foods, especially if the teeth are brushed immediately after eating.

For suggestions for rebuilding jaw bones, see section on Teeth in my forthcoming book, *A New Breed of Patient*.

11. Diabetes

Q. *Recently my family doctor told me that my urine sugar readings were high and advised me to follow a diet eliminating many items in my diet which were staples— i.e., bananas, raisins, honey, grapes—almost all items I believed to be good foods and used. I truly feel a detoxification would greatly aid me and perhaps put me on the road towards good health. Do you have any suggestions?*—A.B., New Shrewsbury, New Jersey.

A. Diabetes is a condition where there is an abnormal metabolism of sugar and fats. To make it simple, there is an excess of sugar in the system which is the result of an insufficient amount of insulin available at the cellular level. I am a firm believer that this condition is partly caused by excessive sugar intake in the diet. This is the same mechanism as the cause of hypoglycemia. Why can the same cause result in two different and diametrically opposite conditions? The only answer I have is that there must be some sort of difference in the genetic factors in the different individuals.

If excess sugar in the diet tends to cause diabetes, we must know a little about the different kinds of sugar involved. First, there are the natural sugars like honey, fruits, molasses, etc. These items do not cause diabetes, in my opinion. However, once diabetes does exist, they may tend to perpetuate the condition. On the other hand, there are the man-made sugars and carbohydrates. These are white sugar, white flour and white rice, mainly. These are items which have been refined by man. In the refining processes, the various associated nutritional factors are eliminated: minerals, protein, fats and other nutrients, leaving only the caloric content.

When these factors have been removed by the refining

78

processes, the body must steal the needed nutrients from itself if they are to be metabolized. This stealing process causes shortages or deficiencies to develop in many areas of the body. When this is done repeatedly, the body finally deteriorates into a state where it must rebel. In this case, we are discussing diabetes, but the mechanism is the same for all disease states.

One of the best approaches to the treatment of diabetes is detoxification followed by rebuilding of the normal structures of the body. I recommend detoxification by the use of mono- or duo-diets. These have been discussed elsewhere in this book (see Hypoglycemia).

Insulin

Q. *I was taught to give myself insulin shots in my upper legs which were well shaped; but now my legs look deformed with deep pockets or indentations where I gave myself the shots. I now give myself shots in my stomach or hips, but my legs have not recovered. Is there anything I can do to get my front upper legs back the way they were—smooth and round?*—D.C., Fort Worth, Texas.

A. Insulin is a very important tool to use in the management of diabetes when all other remedies seem to be of no avail. But, it is quite possible for the body to deteriorate to such an extent that it is impossible to speed recovery by nutritional methods.

Even after all these years of usage, the precise manner of action of insulin evades understanding. There are a plethora of theories but no agreement on which is the truth. I could speculate in your situation that the action of the insulin was direct on the fatty tissue into which the insulin was injected. The reaction caused a breakdown of fatty tissue which then left the empty space you describe as holes. Frankly, this is a very unusual condition and one which cannot be repaired, to my knowledge.

Insulin Shock Therapy

Q. *I was small (size 12), until I was given insulin shock treatments. Now I am a size 22. I have been on so many diets and nothing seems to help. Please, do you have any suggestions?*—V. R., Chicago, Illinois.

A. Insulin shock therapy is used in the treatment of schizophrenia. Other types of shock therapy are used here, too. I am in no position to try to evaluate them separately but do tend to be against them all.

I feel that schizophrenia is a nutritional disease rather than a functional problem. I agree with Drs. Hoffer and Osmond and others who have developed the use of megavitamin therapy for the treatment of this condition. In the megavitamin therapy the emphasis is on large doses of B-3 (niacin), B-6 and Vitamin C.

I do not know why you have developed obesity following shock therapy. I suspect that it is a part of the replacement mechanism whereby the original symptom complex, which was unsatisfactory, is being replaced by overeating. I would not suspect damage to the brain, but an alteration of the metabolic center whereby food is now utilized in a different manner.

A possible form of therapy would be to institute the megavitamin program. I notice that you are doing just this but you are not specific concerning the particular megavitamins mentioned above. Incidentally, I am wholeheartedly against dolomite as a source of calcium and magnesium. It is a form of inorganic minerals which can only be utilized by the body in a very meager manner. Calcium, for example, can only be utilized by the body in an acid form. Dolomite is rock and mineral. It is calcium-magnesium carbonate. Clinically, it appears to cause even more need for calcium than existed before dosage. It is a very insoluble compound. Some forms of dolomite also contain lead.

Juvenile Diabetes

Q. *My daughter, age seven, weighing 54 pounds, has diabetes. She is on a strict diet and also takes 8 units of U-40 insulin each day.*

How can I help her regain her health so that she can again lead a normal life without the use of insulin?—Mrs. C.M.W., Washington, Pa.

A. Diabetes is a metabolic disturbance in which carbohydrates and fats are not metabolized properly. The net result, which is most important, is called hyperglycemia. The blood sugar goes too high and does not return to normal in the usual period of time. Juvenile diabetes is particularly vicious because it simply means that the patient has had the condition for a much greater percentage of his life and thus the bad metabolic habit patterns are more thoroughly ingrained. If diabetes develops later in life, it is usually less severe because the body has certain metabolic habit patterns which, though they are not working correctly, do have a certain normal basis. This backlog of normalcy is lacking in juvenile patients.

What to do about diabetes is a problem which is an individual one. The physician is challenged to make a very complete metabolic analysis to determine all the individual variations. This cannot be ascertained by a simple history, a scanty physical examination and a blood sugar test, or even by a three-hour glucose tolerance test. In this day and age even a 90-minute glucose tolerance test is used to diagnose diabetes. To me this is brevity to the point of absurdity. I know from long experience of using the five-hour, seven-sample glucose tolerance test on a routine basis that one cannot begin to accurately read these tests until all the five-hour response figures are available.

Nutritional treatment of diabetes demands a thorough liver detoxification program, plus a tissue rebuilding effort. If these are successful, then one can expect improvement. More specifically, the patient should consume a good multiple vitamin product which includes all the naturally occurring synergists.

The pituitary and pancreas are two glands which need support, too. The preparations I use are the tissue extracts of these glands (pituitary and pancreas) from beef sources.

The kidney needs support to help to eliminate all the mobilized toxins from within the body. For this I use raw renal tissue extract.*

Finally, a diabetic patient needs extra amounts of B complex. Here again this should contain all the naturally occurring synergistic factors. A B-complex tablet made up by "properly balancing" all the factors as they naturally occur in nature is not enough. This is like taking a watch apart, placing all the parts into a nice little pile and then applying sufficient pressure to squeeze all these items into the same size and shape as the original, putting them back into the case of the watch and expecting it to keep time.

Diabetics can be helped by nutritional measures. Sometimes the benefit is unbelievable, but not always. As with any other situation, one must use common sense.

Diabetic Neuropathy

Q. *I am 49 years old, diabetic, and have been on insulin 10 years. I am a millwright and work with my hands and arms to a great extent, much of it overhead work. My problem is for the past four or five years I have gradually lost strength in my arms to the point where I can only use tools over my head for a matter of a few minutes. Then I must rest. I am now taking 30 mg Prednisone every other day and the doctors seem to think this has arrested the deterioration though they don't expect any improvement. I don't know much about nutrition, but am curious as to whether diet could help this condition; also wonder about vitamin supplements, particularly Vitamin E. I am now taking B complex and C. Any suggestions?*—G.D., Hayward, California.

A. Diabetes is not the simple disturbance of the metabolism of sugar it was once thought to be. It is also a disturbance in the protein and fat metabolism. Everything is included. Even diabetic specialists cannot now agree on a definition of diabetes!

*See Product Information.

In my estimation, it is a generalized manifestation of malnutrition. This also explains why patients deteriorate in many different ways while the diabetes is under control.

You are experiencing one of these areas of deterioration which, at this distance, I presume to be neurological. This is called diabetic neuropathy. It is showing up in your case in the weakness of the muscles. It could also represent vascular insufficiency.

Treatment for this condition should be a complete nutritional approach. The condition may not be easily corrected since you have been ill for a number of years. You have also been taking Prednisone. This substance is a very unbalanced method of trying to replace or supplement the adrenal cortical function. It can do nothing but cause further imbalances, though it makes you feel better in the meantime. It cures nothing, but causes many problems. I do not understand why the whole adrenal cortex extract is not used, which has little or no side effects; but the refined fraction is generally used, which has many side effects and does not cure.

Total stabilization through nutrition means that all the parts of the body are helped to function in harmony by getting the needed nutrients so that the body can be rebuilt metabolically.

High Blood Sugar

Q. Recently I had a complete physical checkup. Everything checked out fine, except the glucose tolerance test. It showed I was slightly diabetic, much to my surprise, as I have been a follower of health foods, and have been well. My age is 57. There is no history of diabetes in our family.

The doctor explained that it seems I have an obstruction in the pancreas, because my blood sugar is high only during the first two hours of the four-hour test. After that it levels off to normal. There is no sugar in the urine, as yet.

Is there anything I can take, dietwise, that would activate the insulin flow to normal? I dread the thought of taking insulin daily.—B.M.T., Pomona, Calif.

A. Diabetes is not always hereditary, so do not count on this factor.

Having high blood sugar during the first hour or two is only indicative of a prediabetic state. In my estimation, it does not mean that you are diabetic. It would also be very important to know the actual number values of your test. What was the level at the fifth hour? You may have low blood sugar then. If this is true, you are then diabetic, or have hypoinsulinism (low level) during the first hours and hyperinsulinism (high level) at a later time. This then, is an extremely unstable condition known as dysinsulinism or diabetogenic hypoglycemia. Any treatment for diabetes would automatically worsen the hypoglycemic situation in the later hours. In my experience, the treatment is almost exactly the same as for the hypoglycemic state. The only real exception is to stress the stimulation of the pituitary gland rather than the pancreas.

The fact that you have used health foods for the past several years does not mean that you cannot develop diabetes. You certainly cannot erase your hereditary factors by diet, nor can you change your past history, sex, age, etc. Nutrition is only one of the factors which determine the type of illness you may develop in the future. True, it is the only one which can be manipulated to any degree and, in reality, is very rewarding when used therapeutically.

Another interpretation concerning your case which must be investigated is the status of the liver. The so-called block of the pancreas may in reality simply be an under-functioning of the liver.

To me, this problem seems basically nutritional in nature. If, after a checkup such as I have suggested, you do apply the basic principles of good nutrition, you should obtain some beneficial results.

Diabetes and Hypoglycemia

Q. *I have a young female friend who not only has diabetes but suffers from Celiac Disease (malabsorption). She has given up with the doctors because she said she is tired of taking drugs. Are there any specific vitamin supple-*

ments for aiding this disease or can you refer her to any good printed material that would give her more insight into her problem?—M. K., Hot Springs Nat. Park, Ark.

A. That is a pretty fancy diagnosis. I would have to see it to believe it. She more than likely does suffer from diabetogenic hypoglycemia or dysinsulinism. It simply means that the blood sugar goes to high levels and appears as diabetes during the first hours of the glucose tolerance test but falls to hypoglycemic levels in later hours of the test. It is very difficult to treat if one is going to attack it from the diabetes point of view. However, it is relatively simple if one attacks it from the hypoglycemic viewpoint. That includes the nutritional viewpoint also. Just get busy on a complete metabolic analysis and start correcting the deficiencies found therein. In due time, as the patient is being treated, the condition gradually disappears.

Another comment about Celiac Disease is that sometimes the blood sugar just drops and does not rise during the GTT test. My question is: how can the blood sugar just drop out of a clear blue sky if some sugar is not absorbed first to cause the hyperinsulin response? Malabsorption is not the name of the game; it must be hyperinsulinism from some cause.

Diabetes and Thyroid

Q. *I have three problems: 1. My hysband has a diabetic condition, supposedly high blood sugar. His doctor advises Dymelar, a timed capsule, to be taken each morning. We also take vitamins every day but lately he says Vitamin B does not agree with him. Could it be that something in the drug conflicts with Vitamin B? He also takes a B-12 shot once a month. He takes lecithin and Vitamin E, etc., regularly.*

2. I burp a lot after meals and I wonder about hydrochloric acid. Would it hurt to try some and see? Would it harm my body if I took it and didn't need it? I realize sometimes a mixture of foods will cause it.

3. I had a thyroid operation 20 years ago. My thyroid seemed to be underactive. A couple of years ago I found it was overactive and was causing me to have a fast heart

beat and too much energy. The doctor said it either meant
another operation which would be dangerous due to the
scar tissue and the only other alternative was to drink ra-
dioactive iodine. I did and it burned out most of it and I
really feel fine. I was frightened when I read the article
about radioactive fallout and thyroid cancer. I take Vita-
mins A, D and iodine-Natural and all the other vitamins.
Could you advise any specific thing I could do?—E.M.S.,
Walla Walla, Wash.

A. 1. All drugs are antimetabolites of one sort or another. This means that they do interfere with normal metabolism one way or another. It could be that the B vitamins are incompatible with the drug.

2. Your continual burping could probably be due to a
shortage of HC1. I would give it a try.

3. Your concern about radioactivity is warranted. The
necessary dosage needed to kill off the undesirable cells is
not enough to kill the normal cells. However, some of the
normal cells are insulted enough so that they can react at
a later date. What is strong enough to kill cancer cells, for
instance, is strong enough to cause cancer in normal cells
at a later date. So now you are exposed to this destructive
force. What can you do to try to protect yourself? Vitamin
C in large doses is a protective substance. So also, is Vitamin F. Fresh, raw foods are protective and so is a normal
nutritious diet according to my definitions. So, maintain
good health to protect yourself.

12. Digestive Disorders

Stomach Distress; Skin Lesion

Q. *I have read so much about the benefits of yogurt, and I enjoy eating it topped with molasses. However, when I eat it like this, I immediately fill up with bloat and am uncomfortable. I do have a digestive problem, but yogurt gives me the most distress of all. And—it makes me more constipated.*

Another problem is a "white patch" on my lower lip, which is termed "precancerous" and is being "watched" by a skin specialist. It is tender and getting larger slowly. What, in your opinion, is the best thing to do to prevent serious trouble?—A.K.P., Bountiful, Utah.

A. It certainly does sound as if you have a digestive problem. Digestion starts in the mouth where carbohydrate food is masticated, is partly digested and then is passed into the stomach. In the stomach the protein element is attacked by the hydrochloric acid-and-pepsin combination. This is accomplished in an acid medium, which is opposite to the alkalinity found in the mouth. The food, after proper processing in the stomach, passes into the duodenum, where it is attacked by the bile and the pancreatic enzymes. This medium is alkaline, as in the mouth.

Yogurt is a very special food. It is a great neutralizer, but the system needs adequate acid to handle it. Apparently you need to add more hydrochloric acid to your stomach secretions.

Regarding your lip problem, it seems that you have a spot of leukoplakia, which is considered a precancerous lesion. Several things can be used to strengthen the local tissue before it gets worse. One is Vitamin F, used both orally and by local application. Vitamin F is arachidonic acid,* the most highly polyunsaturated fatty acid in the human dietary. Another remedy is to apply a compress of

*See Product Information.

Aloe vera to the lesion on a daily basis. Still another possibility is to apply a solution of orthophosphoric acid and phytin.* This latter substance was made for internal usage, but was accidentally discovered to be good for removing warts and some other types of skin lesions. Sometimes it acts as a "vitamin," causing the wart to grow before it dries up.

Leukoplakia is a potentially serious condition and should be watched carefully by your physician, regardless of what else you do.

Digestive Breakdown

Q. *I have so many aches and pains and my stomach hurts and stings most of the time. When I eat, even my rib cage aches and I feel sick to my stomach. My food is eliminated undigested. I have been given blood tests and X rays to locate my problem, but nothing shows up except low blood sugar and lack of calcium.*

The first doctor I went to said there was something wrong in my digestive tract, but he didn't know what. He has given me pills which aren't helping. I am getting weak and worried. I have been taking vitamins—A, B-complex, C—and minerals, but have constant diarrhea. Whatever I eat leaves my body within 12 hours. I have been put on a bland diet by my present doctor, but my health is going downhill—fast!

I also have trembling, chills and am cold a lot, get short of breath after the mildest exertion. I have low blood pressure and my hair is coming out by the handful. Within the last year, little tiny reddish brown specks and a few bigger just red specks have appeared on my arms and body.

Please give me an idea if you can help me. I am desperate.—Mrs. V.S., Madison, Wisconsin.

A. Here is an example of a complete, or at least, almost complete breakdown of the digestion. This represents very serious defect in the patient and she cannot continue to exist in this manner. Naturally, it is a very complex situation and demands a complete metabolic examination.

*See Product Information.

Next, and most important, is to get the digestive enzymes into the system. To start with, hydrochloric acid is a *must*. Even if you could take it by mouth, and you may be able to do so, you probably cannot consume enough. In my experience, I find it quite necessary to administer hydrochloric acid intravenously. The preparation I use is a 1:1000 dilution administered in doses of 10 to 20 cc at one time, using a large syringe and a 25 gr. needle. Daily, tri-weekly, bi-weekly or weekly administration is needed as determined by the reponse of the patient. Incidentally, the HCl should be given slowly or even diluted more than mentioned because it can irritate some veins. No permanent damage results though it may be sore for a few days.

Next, the patient should have pancreatic enzymes administered. Raw pancreatin tablets are a good source of this.* Bile salts are very essential for proper digestion. Frankly, I prefer to use a weak digestive tablet at first because it is so easy to exceed the patient's tolerance for these enzymes and, especially, hydrochloric acid by mouth.

Naturally, along with this basic approach, the rest of the needed vitamins and minerals should be administered as soon as the patient can digest them.

Shortage of Hydrochloric Acid

Q. *Could a person who has an ulcer be deficient in hydrochloric acid?*—R.J.L., Arcadia, California.

A. I am afraid that there is much to be learned in the area of acid-base balance. I do believe that a shortage of hydrochloric acid can or does cause ulcers. It goes something like this: If there is an insufficient amount of HCl in the system, there will be shortage in the gastric secretions. This causes incomplete digestion of the protein complexes of the food. This means there will be an incomplete digestion of nutrients on a tissue level.

If the stomach of the individual is susceptible, the result will be an ulcer. It could be other areas, depending upon individual susceptibility. The ulcer then becomes worse be-

*See Product Information.

cause of the presence of acid on an open wound. Even this does not answer all the questions because some of the patients who have ulcers can and do feel better with the administration of HCl. Mostly they do not. However, by the administration of hydrochloric acid intravenously, these patients soon rebuild their reserve of HCl and are able to begin to digest the proper protein and thus heal the ulcer.

There are some references to the use of HCl in the treatment for almost all conditions in medical literature. Upon examination of these theories, I have come to the conclusion that HCl is very important in therapy. One aspect of my therapeutic program is the use of HCl in the diet and intravenously. This is done almost routinely with few adverse effects.

Hydrochloric Acid and Digestion

Q. When a high-protein-diet indigestion is alleviated by ingestion of glutamic or betaine hydrochloride and enzyme preparations, what organs or glands are involved? Are any particular nutrients helpful?

Are the hydrochloric acid formulas buffered and if so, what are the buffering mediums?

What are cytotrophins and are they compounded synthetically or on an individual basis from the patient's tissue?
—Mr. C.U., Wichita, Kansas.

A. Since indigestion is relieved by hydrochloric acid, then you can be sure that you are in need of this substance. Your stomach is not producing enough acid to digest the food. This is common in the high protein diet even though you may not be aware of it. When you consider enzymes, you are talking primarily about the pancreas. The nutrients I use to treat such conditions: fresh raw diet consisting of fruits, vegetables, nuts and seeds; an abundance of all the basic nutrients which tend to correct ailing bodily function. Sometimes, with continued intake of HCl and enzymes the basic trouble is corrected so that further therapy becomes unnecessary.

To buffer hydrochloric acid would be the same as making it valueless, so it is not buffered.

Cytotrophins are nucleic acid extracts derived or extracted from various animal tissues. They are not synthetic. They contain the tissue type RNA and other nucleic acid items which combine to make up life. The main source of cytotrophins is beef.

Pancreatin

Q. *I have been taking 2,400 mg of pancreatin and ox bile after meals. A friend said he used to take tablets like these and each tablet contained 300 mg of pancreatin plus other enzymes. The label read, "Caution: Do not take if ulcers or other intestinal irritation are present." Was it the pancreatin or the other enzymes that were irritating to the ulcers? I asked this same question of two druggists and one doctor and they did not know.*—Mr. C.J.G., Bonner Springs, Kansas.

A. To the best of my knowledge and experience, there is no contraindication for the use of pancreatin. Ox bile has been implicated in some cases of gastrointestinal diseases, if taken continuously. The tablets which irritated the ulcer probably contained some HCl.

Stomach Problems

Q. *For several years, I have been having stomach problems of various kinds along with fatigue and a cracked tongue. A doctor's prescription helped but didn't clear up the problems. Do you have any suggestions for these problems?*—L.R., Northridge, California.

A. The reaction you describe in your mouth and on the tongue could also exist in the intestinal tract all the way down. It is indicative of Vitamin-B-complex deficiency. If you can correct the cracks in your tongue, you can certainly correct the gastrointestinal tract lesions at the same time. B complex in all forms in generous amounts is indicated.

Duodenal Ulcer

Q. *I've had my gallbladder out for about 10 years. Seven years ago I started to hurt on the right side of my navel and had an operation because the surgeon thought I might have cancer of the pancreas. They found a duodenal ulcer and a hiatal hernia. They said nothing about fixing the ulcer, only the hernia. Do you have any suggestions or nutritional advice I could follow?*—R.B., Westfield, Mass.

A. I subject my patients routinely to what I call the metabolic checkup. This is described in detail in my book *A New Breed of Doctor*. With the accumulation of all this information, one can begin to see where the patient is deficient. Then, some specific nutrients and tissue supplements can be added to a program designed to cleanse the body and then to rebuild it. Each case is individual and unique. What the symptoms are is relatively unimportant except that this is what brings the patient in for help. When the underlying causes are discovered and corrected, many different kinds of symptoms sometimes disappear.

Stomach Ulcers

Q. *Will you be kind enough to tell me some of the principal causes of ulcers of the stomach? What can be done to get relief?*—W.S.G., Fresno, Calif.

A. Stomach ulcers occur when the normal mucosal tissue is broken down in the stomach and an open sore exists. This breakdown does not occur until there is local tissue failure. The mucous membrane cells are not acting in a normal manner and are susceptible to the effects of the normally present hydrochloric acid in the stomach during the digestive processes. This abnormal cellular function could be caused by an insufficient amount of nutrients getting to the cells from the blood supply, that is, by a deficiency in the circulatory system on a local basis. Not enough blood is reaching a given tissue in a given period of time. When this happens, the tissue suffers and breaks down at its weakest point. When enough of the individual cells break down, then the whole tissue areas suffer and an ulcer may develop in the stomach mucosa.

Another cause is related to the amount and type of nutrients arriving at the tissue level in a given period of time, even when the circulatory system is intact and functioning properly. The usual thing is to find a protein or some other major deficiency. Normal tissue integrity cannot be maintained if the protein level in the blood is insufficient. Nor can it be maintained if there is a shortage of hydrochloric acid. This sounds ambiguous because hydrochloric acid excess is supposedly a causative factor in ulcer production and yet hydrochloric acid deficiency is a cause of the ulcer. To get some sense out of this, one must be aware of the timing. It is necessary that the acid be present in the stomach during the digestive processes. It is when this acid in superconcentration lasts well into the postdigestive phases that the acid causes a digestion of the person's own tissues, and the ulcer develops. If there is enough acid at the right time, and for the right period of time, the digestion is adequate and the protein can be digested and absorbed so that it can go to the stomach mucosa for proper maintenance of the tissue.

One other major area that needs to be discussed here is the nervous control of the stomach. The stomach, like all viscera, is controlled by two nervous systems: the sympathetic and the parasympathetic. The former causes the adrenal type, or stimulative type, of reactions which prepare the body to fight or for flight. The latter is necessary to prepare the body for rest and digestion. When these nervous influences are at odds, trouble develops, because the tissues and organs do not know which way to react at which time. Excessive acid can be secreted into the stomach at a time when it is not needed, and not enough when it is needed. Or there can be too much muscular contraction at the wrong time. All these functional actions can be the result of poorly balanced nervous control of the stomach, or the result of emotional problems.

Most stomach ulcers can be treated by the application of basic nutritional efforts designed to strengthen the whole body and, incidentally, the stomach. My usual method of treatment includes a dietary approach consisting of the simplest of diets which can be taken without upsetting the stomach. I try to get the patients to eat only one food for a period of two weeks. This one food is especially adapted for the patient and for the season of the year. The food is eaten at frequent intervals, sometimes as often as every hour. The patient is also given something containing comfrey and mucin or pepsin. To protect the mucous membrane of the stomach from the action of the abnormally concentrated hydrochloric acid, they may be taken on an hourly basis.* When the patient begins to improve, I do not become too anxious to change the routine, because if it takes two weeks to heal a sprained ankle, it must take at least that time to heal an ulcer. This is true even when there are no symptoms. Do not be hasty. Gradually, as one is sure of his ground, the diet can be expanded to include varied foods, many of which may formerly have been troublesome.

Diverticuli and Duodenal Ulcer

Q. *I have found out I have diverticuli in my lower intestines. I love raw vegetable salads but I know it creates lots of gas so I imagine it is not what I should eat even though we should eat raw food. What is your answer?*

Also I would like to know about a duodenal ulcer of the colon. Would colonics be harmful? Would buttermilk or yogurt be good also?—Mrs. O.K., Kennewick, Wisconsin.

A. Diverticulosis is a condition where there are small outpocketings of the mucosal lining of the intestinal tract, especially in the large intestine. Diverticulitis is the condition where the diverticuli are inflamed for one reason or another. This is where there is infection present. Unfortunately, the things you need for a cure are the very things that cause you the trouble. The big secret is how to get these into your system without causing you too much trouble in the process. In the usual medical management, there is no real attempt to correct the condition. They just try to get the condition calmed down, so that you can live with it, by using various types of sedatives and bowel deactivators. The results are usually the same: a state which could

*See Product Information.

get out of control at any moment. Usually the next step is the excision of the colon.

Nutritionally, there are many things that can be done. First, as usual, there must be a complete metabolic survey. This gives many leads as to what your specific problems are and what to do about them. Specifically, the mucosal lining of the intestinal tract must be soothed. A small amount of bran taken daily is the newest Haftes treatment.

Raw foods can be juiced or pureed in a blender. Buttermilk and the right type of yogurt is helpful, too, because it is also wise to reestablish the normal intestinal flora in the tract. This is done also by using the proper acidophilus preparation (found in health stores), and various herbs such as spinach, pineapple, cabbage or the true herbs in the herbal tonic you asked about, which is available through health food stores. Enemas containing these cultures can also be used along with the oral approach. Here you tackle the problem from both ends and the results are forthcoming sooner and more forcefully.

Comfrey and pepsin are great soothers of intestinal mucosa. Hourly dosages may be necessary for control at first.

The duodenal ulcer in the colon sounds like a Meckle's diverticulum which can contain an ulcer. Meckle's diverticulum is a piece of aberrant stomach tissue located in a pouch just proximal to the ilio-cecal valve in the ilium or part of the small intestine. The mechanism is just the same as with stomach ulcers only the location is different. Surgery is required to solve this problem. I do not know of any nutritional approach which would be of real value here.

Inflamed Appendix

Q. *Is there anything that will arrest an inflamed appendix and prevent surgery?*—H. T., New York, N. Y.

A. Colitis is simply an inflammatory condition of the bowel, often including the appendix. This condition does not warrant surgical removal of the appendix. However, if the inflammation is limited to the section of the bowel known as the appendix, the recommended therapeutic choice is surgical excision. If the appendix alone is inflamed, there is a good chance that it will suppurate and cause an abscess. This is not necessarily a fatal condition, but it is certainly one that prolongs convalescence.

What are some of the simple remedies which could help to cause an appendix to subside without removal? One is to use an ice bag on the abdomen and to sip ice chips. Both of these measures act to slow down peristalsis and thus tend to allow the body defenses to build up to a good fighting level. Rest is good, too. Vitamin C in large dosages strengthens the antistress forces in the body. Raw thymus tissue causes a reaction in the endothelial system which increases the body's ability to produce antibodies, and if there is enough time in this illness, they may be of value.*

Hydrochloric acid can help to relieve acidosis in the system. The "good" acid will help to remove the "bad" acids which are an accumulation of metabolic wastes.

Colonic irrigations can be of value in helping to mechanically remove the accumulated toxins in the gut and from the site of the appendix. I do *not* mean an enema. Enemas produce increased pressure and can cause an acute appendix to rupture, whereas the colonic is quite gentle and can be beneficial. *Laxatives should never be taken when appendicitis is suspected.*

All these measures may sound safe, but I will be the first one to advise you not to try them by yourself. You should be under the watchful eye of your doctor when you use them, so that surgical intervention can be instituted immediately if the need is indicated.

Chronic Constipation

Q. *I have been getting severe headaches about once a week. I think that not having enough bowel movements is causing them. I try to do without aspirin, but the pain gets so severe that I become ill if I don't take something to ease the misery. Can you suggest something that would give me good elimination?*—E.A., Lakeside, Calif.

A. Chronic constipation can certainly cause headaches and other signs of toxicity. You can even be constipated

*See Product Information.

while having bowel movements each day. The feces can become packed against the walls of the intestines and stick there even while there is a normal flow in the middle.

I certainly believe in a definite bowel cleansing program under these circumstances. The simplest method is to use repeated enemas, even twice daily until a normal habit is established after each meal. Colonics do a better job, but must be administered by a technician. There are several types of bowel cleansers available on the market.

I am quite sure that if you get good elimination, the headaches will be a thing of the past and you will not need pain pills.

Constipation

Q. *I am 48 years old and since my early years have had a chronic state of constipation. I have tried all sorts of medications for my ailment but have found no results. What do you suggest?*—M. G., San Antonio, Texas.

A. The true and lasting answer to your problem is a raw diet. You will be amazed when you begin to have normal bowel movements after eating nothing but raw foods for a period of time. In the beginning, you must take many enemas to be sure to clean the lower intestine of its accumulated products. Enemas should be taken even twice daily to accomplish this. Do not worry about becoming addicted to enemas because this is not true. Nor will it deplete your supply of nutrients within reason.

The important part here is that you do eat the raw diet while this is going on. Naturally, you need to eat much more volume to get the necessary nutrients so there will be something for the bowel to work on. This is a high fibre diet, but may be enhanced by using a few tablespoons of soft (not rough) bran flakes daily. Sooner or later you will be rewarded.

Impactions of the Intestines

Q. *Please, how does one get rid of the impactions of the intestines after years of lack of hydrochloric acid? This has been definitely diagnosed through iridiagnosis. Enemas and colonics do not help.*—Mrs. H. W., Lancaster, Pennsylvania.

A. My approach to the problem would be to do exactly as you have done: use enemas and colonics. In addition to the mechanical approach I would get as much hydrochloric acid and digestive enzymes into the system as possible. Then, to round out the program, one must have an intake of the bulky foods, raw foods, to have something to push through the intestines. This latter could be assisted by the bulk type bowel conditioners, or a small amount of bran daily. The combination of these approaches should eventually eradicate the bowel impactions.

Colonics

Q. *In your column you mentioned that colonics taken correctly could be of benefit. Could you explain how it is done correctly so that the body is not harmed?*—W.F., Cuernavaca, Mex.

A. Colonic irrigations are a great therapeutic blessing when handled correctly. There are many conditions where the removal of the detoxification products via the bowel is greatly enhanced by this technique. I have even ordered colonics to be taken on a daily basis for a controlled period of time in some extremely ill patients, with great benefit. Other times, it is more sensible to use them on a weekly or semiweekly basis. When they are used in this manner, one does not become "addicted" to them. In fact, normal bowel habits are established in this manner. Many pockets of toxic material can be loosened from the colon, which aids in the detoxification program.

The danger of the colonic irrigation is not, as many assume, that the colon can be ruptured. This is almost impossible because there is less pressure used than in the usual enema. To me, the greatest danger is in the loss of electrolytes. When one uses the colonic it is an in-and-out repetitive cycle which causes the water to slowly loosen and wash out the bound fecal material. In the process of doing this, the "good" electrolytes (minerals) are also pulled from the blood into the bowel to maintain the normal electrolytic balance between the blood and the colon. If the colonics are too long or are too frequent, this is a danger, especially when the patient is already short in mineral supplies. The sudden and acute loss of sodium, for instance, can cause the reaction known as heat exhaustion. In order to overcome this reaction, it is necessary to drink some salt, preferably sea salt, in water, at once. A dosage of one teaspoonful in a glass of water can give benefit to this acute loss of minerals within a couple of minutes.

The colonic has great benefits when used properly, but there may be danger when it is used without proper caution. This is the area where a physician is helpful.

Bowel Reaction

Q. *It is possible to largely or completely eliminate pathogenic bacteria from the intestinal tract by using acidophilus, garlic, etc.? Such bacteria are normally present in everyone, I understand, and do no harm under ordinary circumstances. However, they cause me a lot of harm. My problem is a tendency to rectal abscesses and fistulas. I have been to several doctors and have had surgery twice, but sooner or later, usually in the fall or winter, I get an attack. I have asked these doctors how to prevent recurrences, but they have no answer except to avoid constipation (which I am rarely troubled with, anyway). They have no answer at all as to why I am prone to such infections. Conventional medical opinion is that a rectal fistula cannot heal without surgery because it is continually reinfected by bacteria from the stool.*—G.M., Santa Maria, California.

A. You apparently do have an unusual bowel reaction. In each instance of surgery, they were not able to eliminate all the infection so that a seed remained in the tissues in a different place. Thus, when things go wrong and your resistance is lowered, you develop a recurrent infection.

There are two main avenues of approach. The first is, as you suggested, to flood the intestinal tract with acidophilus bacilli. This should be done as soon as possible and as effectively as possible. I would suggest, as a starter, that Kefir or acidophilus live bacilli in liquid or capsules be taken at bedtime and in the morning before breakfast. This amounts to about one-million count of acidophilus culture, twice daily. The Kefir or yogurt can also be administered rectally, as well as by mouth, as a retention type enema.

Along with this attempt to repopulate the intestinal tract with friendly bacteria one should attempt to strengthen the resistance of the body. I find a good approach is to use the SPL antigen. This is Staphage Lysate. I use an intradermal injection of 0.1cc once weekly for a period of 12 or more weeks, depending upon the response of the patient. This is a slow approach, but very satisfactory in an apparently insoluble problem such as yours.

Problem Bowels

Q. *I have a terrible problem with my bowels. I get gas and feel very bloated—the gas rolls back and forth in the bowels and I can't seem to expel the gas. I have tried many different ways to solve this problem but haven't found an answer. Could you suggest anything for this situation?*—M.P., S.J., California.

A. First of all, you need a bowel cleansing program. The simplest thing is to take one herbal laxative tablet each evening for a month. You are not interested in a large cathartic reaction but a simple stimulation of the bowel. You also need hydrochloric acid. Betaine hydrochloride plus pepsin from the health food store should do the trick. Be sure to take enough to do the job. Too much causes heartburn so you will know when to cut back on that dosage.

You may continue enemas for a while until the bowels begin to move on their own. Since you have been addicted to these and to colonics, I would suggest a strong oral mineral supplementation, especially calcium. In order to get the most out of calcium, it may be necessary to take Vitamin D, too—in large doses.

You probably need more sodium in the system. True, sodium retention does play a part in some diseases but it is also necessary for health. If there is one single thing that I have found, it is a universal lack of sodium. It is the kind of salt and sodium taken that is the problem. True sea salt is the answer but this must be sun dried, as a whole product—not just partially evaporated. Be sure that your product is sea water toally dried out with nothing removed.

Yes, friendly bacteria are important. I advise an acidophilis culture to be taken daily or twice daily. Along with this, one should take whey to ensure a friendly environment for the friendly bacteria.

These are the basic steps to take. You also need all the vitamins, especially B complex.

Paratyphoid and Bowel Problem

Q. *We would like to know if you can come up with a reasonably good natural means of getting over paratyphoid? We have also had typhoid, typhus, brucellosis and one other which I cannot recall at the moment. Our digestive systems are in bad shape now as well due to this infection. We need very desperately some way to bring things back to normal. Do you have any solutions to our problems?*—F. S., Kansas City, Mo.

A. It is rather hard for me to conceive of anyone suffering from typhoid, paratyphoid, typhus and brucellosis and one other as you mention. Even having all these at different times in your life is rather incongruous.

Be that as it may, you apparently do have a bowel problem. First, you need a good basic program. Add to this something like comfrey pepsin to assist in the proper function of the bowel as a means of improving the health of the intestinal mucosa. This can be taken in very large doses, every hour as needed to make the intestinal tract calm down.* I would also consider yogurt, Kefir or other form of acidophilus bacilli. Putting the correct form of bacteria in the intestinal tract can do wonders for the patient sometimes.

I would also consider the use of Staphage Lysate of staphylococcus. It can be used to generate more general resistance in the body. It could conceivably help you to develop antibodies to the paratyphoid and thus eliminate it from your system. Along with this, you could use what I call D & L solution. This is made by adding 1cc of crude

*See Product Information.

liver extract (Lederle or Lilly) and 3½ cc, two percent novocaine to 100cc of pure distilled water containing no
preservatives. The dosage of this is 1cc per 25 pounds
body weight given by injection by your doctor at one time
in multiple sites intramuscularly of not more than 2½ cc
each site.

Rectal Problem

Q. *I have had a rectal problem for the last 15 years or
so (61 now). I have been examined by three local doctors,
the Lahey Clinic in Boston, and a well-known proctologist
in New York, but my problem is still with me. The first
part of my stool is hard and sandy. This causes rectal
bleeding at times and occasionally some hemorrhoids.
What would you suggest for this condition?*—H.L.R.,
Methuen, Massachusetts.

A. Indeed, you have been given the correct advice. You
need more bulk. It is the bulk in the diet which will
reduce the incidence of cancer of the bowel by seven percent. You are also in need of bulk to soften the stool and
to increase the amount so that the bowel has something to
work on. I would urge you to concentrate on the bran and
vegetables rather than the fruits for this material. I also
use comfrey and pepsin.*

One could use a one-ounce olive or sesame oil retention
enema to help start the passage.

Colitis

Q. *Would you please send me any information you
have on colitis?*—R. C., Spring Valley, Ill.

A. That's a big order, especially when you consider that
whole books have been written on this subject.

Colitis is an inflammation of the colon. It can be caused
by allergies, infections or chemical poisonings. One very
important cause would be deficiency diseases. The result of
these on the colon is to cause the local blood vessels to be-

*See Product Information.

come swollen and irritated. This results in an increase in the circulation of the blood to this area. When there is enough congestion of blood, there may be an oozing into the gastrointestinal tract and it may get into the stool. It can progress to the extreme to cause an ulceration of the mucosa of the intestine. It can cause an abnormal production of mucus in the bowel. Mucus accumulations tend to interfere with normal digestion and assimilation of food. The problem is then increased and can result in nutritional deficiencies.

The problem of treatment is to help the inflammation to settle down and get the correct foods into the system via the intestinal tract. This is not so easy because the very foods needed to correct the condition are the ones that often cause symptoms. The big secret is to get the nutritional foods into the system with the least symptom-causing reactions. The solution will vary in each case, but the usually prescribed low residue diet is one lacking the very nutrients needed to correct the condition. It also lacks bulk, which can be fortified by bran intake.

Gallbladder Malignancy

Q. *I have been X-rayed and informed that I have gallstones. This was two years ago. I refuse to be operated on and wish to try nutritional methods to solve the problem. I have heard my condition could become malignant. Is this possible?*—M. L., Voluntown, Conn.

A. Malignancy of the gallbladder is extremely rare, even if stones are present. This is the least of your worries. There are some medical treatments which can be used to good advantage in the treatment of gallstones. The first thing to do is to get the intestinal tract clean by the use of enemas. If one follows the plain water enemas with retention type coffee enemas, it is possible to relax the Sphincter of Oddi sufficiently so that some stones can pass.

The coffee here is to be brewed since the instant types are toxic. A strong cupful of coffee is brewed and then diluted to one pint with water and inserted rectally as a retention type enema. This can yield great relief. Next, I suggest a product made from beet tops.* This substance causes the density of bile to be reduced. When thinner, it flows easier and can easily begin to dissolve or dislodge a stone that causes trouble. Remember, if the stone gets caught on the way out, just use the coffee enemas for possible relief before submitting to surgical removal. Coffee enemas can be used for several days many times daily as needed, all to your benefit.

One can use the following formula: take two ounces of orange or grapefruit or lemon juice and two ounces of olive oil each evening for two evenings. On the third evening double the dose to four ounces each. In the morning after the third evening, a coffee retention enema is to be taken after a cleaning out with a tap water enema.

This is a rather active method for the removal of gallstones. Usually it succeeds but sometimes it does not and surgical relief may be necessary. The important thing here is not to be stubborn but to be wisely alert. If things are not going well and the stone seems to be "stuck," then get help from a surgeon so the delay symptoms can be avoided. There is no real danger here if you do not procrastinate too long before calling for help. Actually, I have to tell you the serious side of the problem, but the odds are very much in your favor insofar as passing the stone without complications.

Liver Detoxification

Q. *You answered a question about ruptured capillaries, suggesting the use of bioflavonoids and a strong liver detoxification program. I would like to know what procedure I would follow for liver detoxification.*—W.W., Richmond, Indiana.

A. Liver detoxification means a process whereby the liver is allowed to resume normal function by the elimination of toxins within itself in order to begin to properly detoxify the blood, the normal function of the liver. It cannot perform these duties when its own cells are congested and full of toxins.

*See Product Information.

How to accomplish this is relatively simple and yet, complicated. First, the load on the liver must be reduced. I do this by advising a very limited diet such as a mono or duo diet for a period of two weeks. The program is to eat the same food or two for a period of two weeks. The choices I usually allow are carrot juice, grape diet, grapefruit-and-celery or pineapple-and-papaya. In addition, I prescribe large amounts of the food supplements.

Other means of detoxifying the liver are fasting, lemon juice and molasses diet and many others. They all arrive at the same place theoretically. My experience has shown me that the method mentioned above is very satisfactory. It is not too drastic so that the patient becomes ill from the program, as on a complete (water) fast.

Exhausted Liver

Q. *I am 41 years old, an engineer, and I have been under considerable stress for many years. My original symptoms: stiff neck, shoulders and wrist. After 14 years, these symptoms were finally relieved by daily yogurt and multiple vitamins with other nutrients, but my stools took on tan color. Pruritis set in. Pins and needles developed. My left foot and leg would fall asleep. Treated with copious amounts of Niacin, Vitamins E and C and shots of ACE, the result was no more falling asleep, but now I have lower back pains with nausea, slight fever, tiredness, insomnia, bloated abdomen.*

I took daily shots of B-12, a weekly shot of B-6, thyroid, ACE, B complex, Niacin, Vitamins C and E, Magnesium, Calcium. Results—pins and needles in both feet and numbness, back pain, fever, bloating, pain in area of liver and spleen, extreme weakness, pruritis, canker sores and absolute dependence on hourly intake of fruit or fruit sugar. Stools still a light tan.

I believe that my liver has been brought to the point of total exhaustion by the various treatments mentioned above as well as by the taking of antibiotics and Butazolidine. If there is any hope to improve my condition, I would guess it would have to be a very gradual approach. Do you have

any advice on how to reverse such a debilitating condition?
—G.K., Indialantic, Florida.

A. In the first place, the spasm of the muscles could
have been due to lack of calcium in the system. One could
also suspect that there was a deficiency of HCl. The
yogurt would increase the acid of the colon which could
have accounted for some improvement as well as the increased utilization of B complex. However, your stool
turned a light tan color. This is exactly what would have
been expected and properly, too. Since there were more
milk type solids in the stool with an abundance of the
friendly bacteria, the stools would naturally turn tan. Then
you developed pruritis which is a sign of B-6 deficiency.
So also was the development of pins and needles in the
feet and legs. HCl and heavy B therapy would have helped
there as well as heavy E dosages to improve the oxygen
situation. Niacin would help here, too, along with pyridoxine (B-6).

Then you developed a state of intestinal toxification.
The food was being incompletely digested which resulted
in fermentation rather than digestion. This causes excessive bloating and gas. The other symptoms would probably
be accounted for on the basis of the intestinal intoxication.
Vitamins E and C would help because of the improved antioxidant activities of both of these vitamins.

Your next endeavor was a hit or miss approach. The B-
12 was supposed to improve the nerve function, also the
B-6, B complex and niacin. These would also improve the
intestinal health, especially of the mucosa or lining of the
intestinal tract. By this time your metabolism was in a
mess.

You certainly do need a complete metabolic examination to determine where and to what extent your problems are. You must certainly follow a special plan which
is organized and has a goal. Hit-or-miss attempts really do
a job sometimes if the problem is not too much out of balance. I would suspect that if one could balance the electrolyte (mineral) status in your body, you would begin to improve in short order. Also HCl should help.

As for the dependence on fruits and fruit sugars for the
rest of your life is concerned, I have found that a diet of
vegetables is much better than fruits. Not that the natural

sugars have caused the condition in the first place but once established, they can be perpetuated by them. Squash and related vegetables have much power in calming one down who is sensitive to fruits.

Regional Ileitis

Q. *I am 19 years old and for four years have been afflicted with regional ileitis of the small bowel. I have taken varying dosages of Prednisolone for three years. The amount now is 10 milligrams a day, but I don't seem to be able to get completely off it. The doctors have described my case as "classic." I have been on a very bland diet for most of this time and have had flare-ups which have sent me to the hospital. Do you have any nutritional advice for me to follow?*—L.N., Bellevue, Washington.

A. Regional ileitis is one condition which usually responds to nutritional methods. Many times this clinical condition is the result of allergic reactions to certain foods. Maybe there are parasites present. Usually we just cannot put our finger on the cause of the condition.

The first order of businesss is to soothe the bowel. For this, I use a comfrey and pepsin product.* I use as much of this material as is needed to control symptoms. This could be as high as two capsules hourly. Along with this I use a nonstress diet. This is NOT a bland diet! It does include one food, as a rule. This food should be well tolerated by the patient and should be raw. This diet is continued along with the comfrey pepsin for a couple of weeks or a little longer. When the symptoms are sufficiently controlled, then other foods are added slowly. Again these foods should be raw. A person can live on two or three foods for a long period of time. As soon as possible, I add the various vitamins.

*See Product Information.

Diarrhea

Q. *My wife, who is 55 years of age, has diarrhea and has had it for more than two months. My wife and I both think that she can be healed through a proper nutritional regimen. Her doctor here is not trained to think in these terms. Could you give any suggestions we might follow to help cure her diarrhea?*—J.K., Escondido, California.

A. The first thing that comes to my mind is the lack of the B complex. Diarrhea is one of the cardinal symptoms for B deficiency. In the treatment with this vitamin, it may be necessary to use the injectable form first. I know that this is a synthetic approach but here I use the vitamins as drugs to conquer the acute phase and then begin to rebuild the intestinal tract by the administration of natural substances. A preparation of comfrey and pepsin* is very valuable in coating the intestinal lining and thus reducing the irritation.

Another cause could be an allergy. This includes the allergic reaction to the chemicals in our environment these days. Not only foods eaten where there may be an unexpected concentration of DDT or some such in the leaves of the lettuce, etc., but even the aromas of chemicals can elicit this reaction in certain individuals. One patient of mine and her son were incredibly poisoned by breathing paint fumes. Their condition resulted in severe discogenic back disease which forced the son to wear a brace for many months. It also caused the mother to have surgery for the attempted correction of the condition in the neck and back at least three times.

Coated Tongue

Q. *I have had a coated tongue for two years and have tried to correct it by my diet, but have not been very successful. At times the coating gets quite thick. I have tried to eat fruits, but it makes my joints and muscles ache. I also take a tablet of hydrochloric acid with bile salts. I do not have any pain or soreness in the region of the liver.*

*See Product Information.

This puzzles me. I wonder if you could suggest something that I should be doing or something I shouldn't be doing?—M.D., Hollywood California.

A. You are on the right track. It is just a matter of taking enough hydrochloric acid. It may also be a matter of the product used. Some are more efficacious than others. It may be especially necessary to take yours with pepsin, too. On the other hand, my favorite solution is one that contains potassium salts in dilute hydrochloric acid.* Another reputedly good preparation is one prepared with pectin. Maybe you need two or three different kinds of hydrochloric acid. The betaine form seems to be the most commonly accepted though glutanic acid hydrochloride does a very good job. Do a little more experimentation and searching.

Halitosis

Q. *I have a problem which I am self-conscious about: Halitosis. I always have a flat taste in my mouth. I have tried various things but to no avail. Do you have any suggestions?*—A.G., East Orange, New Jersey.

A. Halitosis is a common problem. It can be caused by all sorts of oral pathology, by certain lung conditions, usually associated with a chronic condition. It can also be caused by other types of nasopharangyeal problems.

However, by far the most common cause of the condition of halitosis is located in the gastrointestinal tract. Dyspepsia is a very common source of halitosis. Constipation is another. Many chronic diseases of the gastrointestinal tract can and do cause halitosis.

The most important single thing which tends to correct the condition more than any other in my experience is the use of hydrochloric acid. This can be administered both orally as well as intravenously. In the latter situation, I use a 1:1000 dilution of hydrochloric acid intravenously very routinely in my practice.

Another help is to take concentrated, defibered alfalfa tablets, or chlorophyll in some form. Both are body cleansers, and have helped various types of halitosis.

*See Product Information.

Bad Breath

Q. *I am really embarrassed. I have extremely bad breath and an almost constant burning, bitter, putrid taste in my mouth. Tooth X rays show no abscesses, but I wonder if there could be infection in the roots. Or could this be caused by the liver or kidneys—or perhaps emotions?*—Mrs. R.W., Seattle, Wash.

A. Halitosis can be caused by dental and oral problems. However, there are causes of bad breath other than the oral and dental conditions. Usually, I find that there is a disturbance in the digestion, often the liver. It then behooves us to correct the liver function. Sometimes it is the kidneys that are not functioning properly.

In general, the liver (including the bowel), the kidneys, the skin and the lungs are the excretory glands of the body. If there is a disturbance in one of these glands, the others become overworked in trying to compensate for the lack. When the skin begins to over-function, the patient develops body odor. This is because of the abnormal kinds of elements in the perspiration. When the lungs are doing extra work because of liver or kidney disease or under-function, then an abnormally strong breath is noted.

Halitosis is a major complaint demands a complete medical and nutritional checkup and evaluation of the body as a whole, as well as appropriate dental and oral evaluations.

Lack of HCL

Q. *I am under a doctor's care for hypoglycemia. I receive weekly adrenocortical shots plus B-complex shots weekly. I am on a high protein diet.*

I have had severe gas and stomach pains. Through testing it was found I am lacking in enough enzymes or may I say the type of enzymes for digesting milk or any milk products. Vitamins and minerals also cause pain in my stomach. We tried all different brands of vitamins and nothing helped. As a result the doctor took me off all vitamins except Vitamins E, A, D, and C. As a result I eat a lot of meat, eggs, nuts, salads and vegetables. I am about 20 pounds overweight.

I feel better, but my stomach pains and gas still flare up at times. My hypoglycemia is better but I still tire quickly, and need a nap every day. I just can't do what I want to do. My legs get weak and I have to rest.

The doctor says I need vitamins desperately. How can I take vitamins, even yeast, if it causes much pain and gas? My doctor doesn't seem to know what else to do. I also take glutamic acid hydrochloride with each meal.

I should add I am 44 years of age, female, married, mother of two children and stay home. Please can you help me?—Mrs. B.N., Oakhurst, N.J.

A. You probably need more hydrochloric acid. This is the best form because it is natural and occurs in the body. You could also satisfy acid need by using apple cider vinegar. Gradually increase the dosage of HCL until you get results. Then continue the dosage until it becomes too much, which it will do eventually, then cut it down to the point of tolerance. This will be your needed dosage. It could be that you do not need any supplementation at that point.

At the present time because you are consuming a high protein diet, more than likely there is not enough acid to adequately digest the food.

Crohn's Disease

Q. *My son suffers from ileitis (Crohn's Disease). It was diagnosed as such last July, but he has had the same symptoms for almost a year prior to this. He is 29 and his work is in law enforcement, so he is always under stress. I know he needs better nutrition than what has been recommended, but I don't know exactly where to begin.*—Mrs. B.R., San Francisco, California.

A. This is a condition where the terminal 12 to 14 inches of the ileium becomes scarred following a chronic inflammation. It frequently leads to intestinal obstruction. This was one of President Eisenhower's illnesses. The usual treatment from the orthodox viewpoint is surgical removal of the offending segment of bowel. The patient can get along without the section that has been removed. It is rather an expensive manner to control the illness, however.

From the nutritional viewpoint, there are several things that can be done advantageously. Dietary control is a must. Unfortunately, the very foods which will tend to cure the condition are the very foods which will tend to aggravate it. Thus, it becomes a problem to get the correct items into the system without stirring up a hornet's nest.

I would start by finding some sort of fresh, raw food which can be consumed without causing symptoms. I would suggest carrot juice or bananas or avocados or papaya or watermelon, or grapes or several other fresh, raw foods. It is not necessarily true that anyone who suffers from ileitis can consume these foods, but with a little experimentation, one of these foods can be found that will not cause symptoms. When this food is found, it is to be consumed at least every two hours and nothing else for a couple of weeks. At the end of this time, the diet can be expanded to other simple foods which do not cause symptoms.

Hyperacidity

Q. *My problem is gas from indigestion at night. There is no sour stomach, no discomfort from meals, although if I drink a glass of water about four hours after a meal, I can belch gas. Antacids seem to have no effect if taken during the night or if taken three to four hours after a meal. If taken at other times they seem to be a disadvantage. At night I can sleep two or three hours, then get up and drink water (warm is better) then belch out the gas. Then two to three hours more, etc. The only discomfort is from distention in the stomach and intestines. I have tried water fasting and the condition is much worse. With only fruit or fruit juice it is slightly better than with water, but much worse than when eating.*—L.W.M., College Place, Washington.

A. It sounds like you do have an honest-to-goodness case of hyperacidity. It is really a rarity to find one since the popularization of the antacid craze. According to the radio and TV commercials, the antacid is the thing. On a practical level, at least nine out of ten people who take antacids and do get relief, really need acid rather than antacid. The antacid actually causes the secretion of more acid so that the stomach empties.

In your case, the situation seems to be different. A natural way of control would be to drink a large glassful of water just before eating. Also, drink more water to get relief from the disturbance even after meals. Theoretically, this will give you time to get on a good and balanced diet to help the body make its own repairs so that proper stomach secretions will result.

Enzymes

Q. *After six months of trying different remedies for an acute flatulence problem, I found relief using digestive enzyme tablets. This was quite surprising in that a medical examination just prior to the start of my flatulence showed that my enzyme levels were excellent. However, the same examination revealed a urinary infection for which two antibiotics were prescribed and I suspect that my enzyme dysfunction may have been a side effect caused by the drugs. Do you know of any means of restoring normal enzyme activity? I am also taking therapeutic doses of the B and C complexes and eat a lot of yogurt, citrus fruit and other raw fruits and vegetables.—G. V., Las Vegas, Nev.*

A. Certainly drugs and antibiotics can destroy enzymes. How to restore normal enzyme activity is another story. The best way to accomplish this is to eat vital foods—those in which the enzymes have not been destroyed. Next, take vitamins that also contain the naturally occurring enzymes. Then would come enzyme preparations. Now there are many different kinds of enzymes so just taking enzymes may not be the answer. However, it does seem that the enzymes in general are restored within the body when all sorts of vegetable type enzymes are consumed like those found in papaya and pineapple. This is one type of tablet which is dispensed from a drug store or from a health food store.

Hemorrhoids

Q. *Is there any natural way to shrink hemorrhoids, or is there a diet that can help me? My friends tell me there is no natural way.*—A.F., Flushing, N.Y.

A. Hemorrhoids are the evidence of liver disease and the major approach to this problem would be a good liver detoxification program. I say "program" because, in order to adequately stimulate the liver, there must be a multiple approach. The liver does some 300 different jobs in the body. It can be stimulated from many different directions simultaneously.

Collinsonia (root) capsules* are excellent for the stimulation of the healing of the hemorrhoidal veins. In the case of varicose veins, which like hemorrhoids indicate liver problems, collinsonia capsules are also effective.

Crohn's Disease

Q. *I would like to know if you could give my wife some information on Crohn's Disease. It started after pregnancy. She also took the birth control pill after pregnancy. She suffers with diarrhea and terrible cramps. She is on dietetic treatment of the spastic or irritable colon. Also the medication she takes is Prednisone (5 mg—2 tablets four times a day for five days) then discontinues that and goes on Salazopyrin (1 tablet 3 times a day) and continues this until the diarrhea and cramps start again and then goes back on the Prednisone. She is so terribly rundown and thin that she tried taking multivitamins and Vitamin E on her own, but it seemed to go right through her. She asked her doctor about it and he said she should not take them and started to give her iron shots.—Can you give us any suggestions?*—G.A., Courtenay, B.C., Canada.

A. Crohn's Disease is another name for regional ileitis. It is a very difficult condition to treat. I would first put your wife on a diet of some raw juice—she can digest one

*See Product Information.

that would be very soothing and yet very nourishing. Carrot juice or grape juice could be the answers here. It is possible that the first attempt could be a failure. That is OK. Just back up, and charge again. I would also give a special comfrey-pepsin preparation* which is very soothing to the lower intestinal tract.

After this approach is used for a long enough period of time to ensure some degree of healing of irritated intestinal mucosa, then the dietary can be expanded. I would add only one food at a time and do so only on a weekly basis for a while. Avocado would be one of the first foods added since it, too, is very soothing. Further additions can be by choice of the patient, but should not include any cooked foods, particularly the foods considered to be the bland diet usually prescribed by orthodoxy. Gentle treatment for a considerable time are the key points to treatment of regional ileitis.

Coffee Enemas

Q. *I have read that coffee enemas are good for detoxifying the liver. I can't understand why this is so. Isn't there something less harmful that would give the liver the same impetus?*—Mrs. L. J. McC., Des Moines, Ia.

A. This question has occurred to me many times, too. I have not come up with an adequate answer as yet. An important fact to consider is that when one uses this type of action, there is great need and the patient is in trouble. I have recommended the use of brewed coffee enemas for individuals who have a history of acute liver or gallbladder colic. Many times the acute problem has subsided even before I could get to the patient for more definitive help.

When coffee is absorbed from the rectum, it is taken into the blood, which then, normally, passes directly to the liver. It appears that the caffeine in the coffee is responsible for the direct stimulating action, but I do not know this for certain. Coffee taken by mouth is absorbed in the stomach and, as such, bypasses the liver in the concen-

*See Product Information.

trated form. This is why coffee taken orally does not have the same action on the liver as the coffee enema.

Meanwhile, the patient is instructed to have a complete analysis and to embark on a total nutritional program.

13. DMSO

Q. *What is DMSO good for? Is it now on the market? Is it harmful?*—E.C.H., Vancouver, Washington.

A. The answer to this question is found in a pamphlet published by Independent Citizens Research Foundation for the Study of Degenerative Diseases, Inc., 468 Ashford Avenue, P.O. Box 97, Ardsley, New York 10502.

DMSO is Dimethyl Sulfoxide, a colorless liquid derived from lignin, the cement substance in the wood fiber of trees. It has practically no toxicity in animals or men. It has been used for arthritis, both osteo and rheumatic types, burns, eyes (herpes edema; uveitis), frozen shoulder, headache, both vascular and tension, interstitial cystitis, injuries, herpes zoster (shingles), osteomyelitis and scleroderma.

It appears that DMSO is a political football. It seems to be one of those things that is not supposed to be available to the public. I can only speculate as to why. There is a book now available which tells the DMSO story. It is called *The Persecuted Drug, The Story of DMSO,* written by Pat McGrady, Sr., and published (1973) by Doubleday.

DMSO Treatment

Q. *I read your answer to the question referring to DMSO. It was very informative and offers hope for the arthritic. I have rheumatoid arthritis and have tried every drug on the market and physical therapy, but continue to have progressive crippling and pain. I am now trying nutritious meals with vitamins and mineral supplements and yet have low grade anemia and crippling. Kindly refer me to a doctor who would apply DMSO for treatment. I have*

117

been told it has to be applied under the most sterile condi-
tions. Is this true? Please tell me the side effects of "gold
shots."—Willis, Texas.

A. My knowledge and experience concerning DMSO is
minimal and limited to hearsay evidence only. I have
never used this substance in my practice. I am led to believe that this substance does assist in the alleviation of arthritic discomfort by simple application and massage to
the local area. It works in minutes, but must be reapplied
after a period of time. No sterile technique is needed.
There seem to be no contraindications to its use, nor does
it cause any side effects of consequence. It is one of those
ideal situations where results are obtained with minimal
risk.

At present, this item is a political football. The "ins" are
against the freedom of use of this preparation. It is being
studied in the great universities under "lock and key." For
information on this timely subject, send a small or large
contribution to: Independent Citizens Research Foundation, 468 Ashford Ave., Ardsley, New York 10502. They
will send you a brochure which is well worth the $1 asked.

Gold is one of the heavy metals. As such, it can cause
all the complications that are caused by other heavy
metals. These complications include blood, bone and liver
disturbances. While taking gold injections, you must be
watched closely. This is so the gold can be discontinued if
side effects become too great. This is the same old story of
closing the barn door after the horse is gone.

14. Drugs

Drug Side Effects

Q. *Please tell me what foods and liquids and vitamins will help a person who took too many diuretic tablets by mistake*—Mrs. E. O'D., Syracuse, N.Y.

A. How did you take too many diuretics by mistake? Did you take them all at once or did you take them in too large a dosage for too long a period of time? There are a couple of points which should be known. For answering purposes, I am assuming that the mistake was in taking the tablets over a long period of time. The major complication in such a situation is the disturbance in the sodium and potassium concentrations within the body.

These deficiencies can be manifested in various ways, but the treatment is the same. The need is to replenish the supply of these minerals as soon as possible. This is why, sometimes, the injection of salt and potassium solutions into the vein can be a lifesaving treatment. If time permits, the administration of these minerals by mouth will usually control the situation.

I usually approach this problem in a multiphasic manner. First, I have the patients drink water containing sea salt (¼ teaspoonful in a glassful of water) once daily, or maybe twice, for a period of two weeks. Along with this, I have them take a tablet containing alkaline trace minerals. In addition to this, I have patients drink "Big Gee Gee" raw sugar cane syrup, which is high in these same minerals (2 teaspoonfuls daily in 1 glass of water). Additionally, the acid content of the stomach is enhanced by the use of apple cider or wine vinegar, three or four tablespoonfuls in water with each meal.

All of these approaches are aimed at the correction of mineral balance within the body. Under the circumstances, there is no fear of using sodium (found in sea water). Sodium has been greatly abused in medical thinking. Sodium is necessary for proper mineral action within the body.

B and C vitamins are also washed out of the body by diuretics. Since they are water soluble, adding them through the use of supplements and brewer's yeast and liver should help.

Tranquilizer Aftereffects

Q. *I've been taking the tranquilizer Librium in the 25 mg dosage for twelve years, usually just one a day. With the doctor's advice I'm now off of it completely. In one week's time, I have undergone many withdrawal symptoms. Scalp sensitivity, extreme excitability, compulsive eating and sensitivity to noise. My nervous system is all out of order. I haven't been able to sleep well either. From a nutritional view point what would you recommend?—A.H., Cincinnati, Ohio.*

A. There are two substances your body needs desperately at this time. First, B complex, especially the B-3 or niacinamide. I would suggest the natural B complex along with about 2000 mg of niacinamide. If this is insufficient, it can be increased. But do not increase the dosage too rapidly. If you are consuming a balanced and optimal intake of the various vitamins, I am sure you will not have to resort to such extreme dosages.

The second substance needed is calcium. I would use raw bone meal* for this. To this you may add extra magnesium and silica. These two elements seem to help the utilization of calcium in the body. It is also necessary to have an adequacy of sodium in order to absorb calcium properly. Sodium can be taken either in natural filtered sea water, or *whole* sea salt, both from health stores.

Tranquilizers

Q. *I have been on a maintenance dosage of Sinequan—55 mg a day for several months. Although I have*

*See Product Information.

tried discontinuing, I find I still need it chiefly for getting to sleep. I wish to do without this drug as it deadens my alertness slightly and, to a greater extent, reduces my energy. Could you please give me specific suggestions as to how to use vitamin therapy for my needs?

A. In this day and age, we consume sedatives, tranquilizers and aspirin, nationally, by the ton each day.

Drugs are used to manipulate the body so that a temporary desirable reaction takes place. It does *not* solve the cause of the problem, and eventually creates serious side effects.

If one wishes to correct the cause of the problem, the body must be rebuilt and supported in all areas of function. This is done by feeding the body all the nutrients needed for normal function of the various parts. If the metabolism of each cell is normal, then the whole body functions normally. It is as simple as that, but this philosophy is utterly ignored by the orthodoxy. Many conscientious doctors cannot see this simple truth. Just talk to a breeder of prize dogs or thoroughbred horses and see how much they value proper nutrition for health. This applies to humans, too.

Ritalin

Q. *Exactly what is Ritalin and how does it work on the brain? Are there any undesirable side effects or reasons that it should* not *be taken? Wouldn't a good megavitamin therapy be preferable for a nervous child with hyperactivity?*—Mrs. M.C.L., Eureka, California.

A. Ritalin is methylphenidate hydrochloride and is used as a stimulant to treat narcolepsy, drug-induced lethargy, and other forms of hypoactivity (under-activity). Strangely, Ritalin acts as a stimulant for adults; but a depressant for hyperactive children. It is used rather extensively in our schools today, sometimes even without the knowledge of the patients. It can overstimulate the individual.

Frankly, I disagree with the whole philosophy of treatment of school children by this method. My experience tells me that if these children were given an adequate nutritional breakfast each and every morning, they would soon be able to think according to their normal ranges. It is easy to judge the nutritional intake of pupils by the grades they get and, vice versa, to predict the accomplishments to be attained by the pupils by determining the food intake at the beginning of the semester. Good food makes healthy bodies and sound minds. I know that there are certain congenital and birth defects which cannot be categorized, but sometimes a good nutritional program will develop a student's potential.

I do not agree with the entire megavitamin concept. In this concept, most vitamins used are the synthetic type. True, they do help, but the real improvement occurs when the food or truly organic vitamins are also taken. The reaction from this natural program is more lasting and more gentle for the patient. However, I sometimes do use the megavitamin ritual when the need is urgent.

Steroid Drugs

Q. *I have just read an article which states that the taking of steroid drugs will cause diabetes. Have you any information on this?*—J.P., Rock Springs, Wy.

A. Steroid drugs or hormones are those secreted by the adrenal cortex glands. They are forms of these hormones which are not the same as the whole adrenal cortex extract (ACE). The latter contains all the naturally present hormones in the concentration as found in the gland. There are absolutely none of the usual complications to the administration of ACE as there are with the administration of the steroids. One of the many and numerous serious complications to the administration of steroids is diabetes mellitus. Pituitary type reactions are also some of the common complications to the overdosage of steroid therapy. Osteoporosis, mineral disturbances and many others are usual complications. Sad but true, the orthodox medical opinion believes that the use of whole ACE is obsolete, and that the use of the steroids is the "in" thing to do and that no one should do otherwise. I do not agree!

Tetracycline

Q. *I am working in a health food store and have been asked by a client about the drug, tetracycline. Before this individual became interested in the health foods, he was affected several times with a prostate infection. For this, his doctor prescribed tetracycline for a 10-day period. The infection returned twice after six months of treatment. He would like to follow a diet which will prevent the infection from recurring, but the main question is: What effect does this particular drug have on the body and how can he, at this point, supplement his diet to help remove or protect himself from the side effects?*—H.K., Tsawwassen, B.C., Canada.

A. Tetracycline is the generic name for a whole series of compounds produced by several different drug houses. It is one of the antibiotics. Antibiotics are divided into two classes: bacteriocidal and bacteriostatic. The former means that the drug will kill the bacteria while the latter term means that the drug will only stun the bacteria. This little point makes all the difference in the world since a dead bacteria will no longer be a problem but a stunned bacteria will eventually return to full vigor and action unless the body is able to mobilize added strength and resistance to thoroughly wipe out the stunned organisms.

In my experience, I have found that the use of the bacteriostatic (stunning) drugs was a waste of time in the great majority of cases; there was quite frequently a recurrence of the problem within a certain period of time. In other words, the infection was not cured, only temporarily made better. For instance, one local doctor used to use a dosage of the tetracyclines at the rate of one four times daily. He would order only six capsules—one and one-half days' supply. The patient usually felt better by that time but was sick again within a week or ten days. It was then necessary to get another prescription for another batch. You are aware of what this means when a doctor gains control over a patient so that he is compelled to return for further care.

When I have to use an antibiotic (and I still do when caught in a bind) I use penicillin which is bacteriocidal (bacteria killing) and thus solve the problem then and there.

15. Ear Problems

Vasomotor Instability and Ear Infections

Q. *Whenever I experience any emotion such as joy, excitement, fear, nervousness, etc., whenever I am out in the hot sun, when I'm dressed too warmly, or in a too warm room, my skin (especially on the face, neck, chest and upper arms) gets these awful red blotches. The blotches are not raised and they burn. Also, I've had much pain during my 38 years with ear infections and irritations and clogging of the eustachian tubes. Do you have any suggestions for these problems?*—B.B., Knoxville, Tenn.

A. You are suffering from a certain type of vasomotor instability. It is rather common, especially in allergic type individuals with fair skin. What to do about it is another question.

Chronic ear infections and congestion are many times allergic in origin. However, by the time they have existed for many years, they probably become infectious. The most common organism found in such a case would be the staphylococcus.

For this condition, I would recommend SPL or Staphage Lysate.* The use of 0.1cc intradermally once weekly for at least 12 weeks and many times many more weeks, depending upon response.

Mechanically one can manipulate the Eustachian tube. The tube can be probed less severely without an anesthetic in conjunction with the balloon treatment of the nasal passages. This causes a popping of the bones just as you get the kinks out of your neck or back after a hard day. This treatment is very simple but should be done by an expert.

*See Product Information.

Tinnitus

Q. *Since March of 1972, I have developed a buzz in the left side of my head and I can't seem to get rid of it.*—Mrs. M.R.A., Monrovia, California.

A. It sounds like you have developed tinnitus in the left ear. This is a condition where the nerves of the ear transmit impulses which are registered in the brain as noise. The impulses may originate from many different causes. First, there may be hardening of the arteries in proximity to the ear so that the noise of the blood rushing past the ear is picked up and transmitted to the brain as noise. This type of tinnitus is intermittent, corresponding to the beat of the heart or pulse wave as it passes the ear.

Another form of tinnitus is due to the irritation of the tiny receptor nerves in the cochlea or part of the inner ear. Depending upon which nerve fibers are stimulated, the noise heard is of a certain pitch. Another type of tinnitus is caused by infection within the cochlea. Naturally, this presents an acute emergency but I do not think that you qualify here.

Another type is the result of loss of integrity of the nerve tissue. For instance, Vitamin B complex deficiency can cause the nerve to act strangely. The auditory nerve is no different from any other nerve in the body. It is my opinion from your description that you are suffering from the B complex deficiency type of tinnitus. This means to get busy with Vitamin B intake. The dosage of whichever member is involved may be very high. Your need may be many times the "Recommended Daily Allowance" like maybe 5 mg folic acid three times daily for six months or so to get results. Other members of the B complex have to do with nerve integrity also, so maybe the whole complex should be taken in large quantity. B-12 must accompany folic-acid therapy.

Ménière's Syndrome

Q. *What can be done to relieve Ménière's syndrome? My ears ring, I have nausea and headaches with an aching sensation.*—B.G., Willis, Texas.

A. Ménière's syndrome is a condition of the inner ear where abnormal noises may be heard or the balance may be disturbed so that one is troubled with vertigo, nausea, vomiting and tinnitus a good deal of the time. In natural treatment there are a few things that can be done. One is to stimulate the circulation to the middle ear, and maybe the inner ear, by pulling on the ears, strangely enough. The more nutrients that can be taken to the area, the more waste products will be removed.

The technique is to put the thumb into the external ear canal. Grasp the lobe of the ear with the index finger. Firmly raise the ear upward under steady tension. Then with a firm "j"-like pull, pull the ear forcefully down and outward away from the head. It is usual to hear a pop of the eardrum. This opens the middle ear and Eustachian tube. Putting your ears through this exercise on a daily basis can improve your abnormal buzzing and dizziness. It could also help the hearing in some cases. One of my cases was a former soldier who had experienced buzzing in the ears since active service when he was exposed to the shattering sounds of heavy artillery. Daily exercises enabled him to hear better as well as to relieve the tinnitus.

You should also embark on a *total* nutritional program. Ears are only one representative of the entire body and its metabolism, but if metabolism is erring in one area, is is also erring in another or on the verge of doing so.

Dizziness

Q. *I have been plagued with dizzy spells when I sleep at night and on arising in the morning. My doctor says my trouble is "vertebral basilar artery insufficiency" in my head.*

I am taking four Arlidin (six mg) tablets a day (for

seven months), but I'm not improving. Can you recommend a diet or supplements that will help me?

Also, what is "Friedreich's ataxia" and what is the cure, if any?—M.S.T., San Diego, Calif.

A. Friedreich's (or hereditary) ataxia is an inherited disease, usually beginning in childhood or youth, with sclerosis of the dorsal and lateral columns of the spinal cord. It is attended by ataxia, speech impairment, lateral curvature of the spinal column, with paralysis of the muscles, especially of the lower extremities.

Dizziness or vertigo at night and upon arising in the morning sounds like a problem of the vestibular apparatus in the inner ear. This is your equilibrium center and it can cause peculiar symptoms with the changes in position of the head which occur in turning over in bed or on arising. In my opinion, this is a nutritional problem. The first approach I would use would be to detoxify the liver. The various glands would need to be supported, and the dietary intake must be adequate not only for nourishment from day to day but also to cause healing. This demands an excess of all nutrients to be available at all times. If there is also "vertebral basilar insufficiency," I would concentrate on the intake of lecithin, polyunsaturated fatty acids, Vitamin B-6 and bioflavonoids, plus a good general vitamin, mineral and enzyme intake.

This may also result from radioactive fallout. Sodium alginate (from health stores) helps to neutralize the effect.

16. EDTA

Q. *I read about the use of EDTA, a chelating agent which literally draws the calcium out of hardened arteries and arthritic joints. Since I have rheumatoid arthritis and have calcification of the finger joints, I wish to know more about this substance. What guidelines can one use to know who is competent enough to use this procedure? What side effect can one expect when receiving this treatment?*— Mrs. L.H., Willis, Texas.

A. Since EDTA (an abbreviation for ethylene-diamine-tetra-acetic acid) is a relatively new therapy, I guess there will be many and repeated questions concerning it. EDTA is a chelating agent. It is administered intravenously so that the chelating effect is directly on the calcium of the blood, as well as some other electrolytes. EDTA binds the metal so that it is excreted through the urine. Then, since the chemical equilibrium of the calcium is disturbed, more calcium is mobilized from the tissues—in the usual case, the arteries which have been hardened. Or the bursa, or the joints (I am not sure about rheumatoid arthritis, but probably osteoarthritis), etc. The conditions are usually helped but one must be careful of possible complications of too much calcium and other electrolytes (minerals) being removed from the system and the possibility of having some of these materials being deposited in the kidneys. Kidney damage is a definite complication which must be guarded against. As with any treatment, one must weigh the good against the bad.

How to establish the competency of the doctor administering EDTA is a good question. I am acquainted with a group of doctors who are working hard to define these terms. They are setting standards of pretherapy care that must be rendered, the conditions that are considered treatable, the term of treatment, the emergency equipment that should be immediately available and any other sort of question that comes to mind, including a certain minimal degree of training and study to be accomplished by the physician. This group is now officially organized: Academy of Medical Preventics, Suite 700, 350 Parnassus Ave., San Francisco, Cal. 94117.

17. Eye Problems

Problem with Vision

Q. *I am a woman 57 years old, 5 feet, 4 inches tall and weigh 155 pounds. I have trouble with my right eye. Something which resembles a black cobweb seems to be floating in front of it. What is this, and what causes it? What can I do about it? It is very annoying.*—C.S.S., St. Louis, Mo.

A. It sounds as if you have a floater in the vitreous of the eye. This is the chamber just in back of the lens of the eye and contains a vitreous substance, something like jelly. This chamber comprises the largest part of the eye. It is through this substance that the light rays pass before they fall upon the retina to create the image. The vitreous humor is very static and not subject to change. That is to say, not subject to normal change. An abnormal change, like a hemorrhage into this chamber, can cause blindness if it includes a large enough amount of blood. If it is only a small amount of blood, then varying degrees of visual disturbance can result.

You apparently have a small amount of hemorrhage, maybe even one blood cell floating in the direct pathway of the light rays. It is located in a critical spot and that is why it bothers you. Once it is "put into orbit" in the vitreous, it does not change position. That is why the spot of distortion always seems to be in the same place. There is no way of getting this foreign body out of the vitreous substance without damaging the eye permanently. Vitreous does not reform, and thus it cannot be tampered with without causing permanent eye damage.

About the only constructive thing that you can do is to guard against possible further damage. Hemorrhagic diseases are felt to be the result of deficiencies of bioflavonoids and other members of the C complex. I would certainly recommend abundant intake of the C complex, including the bioflavonoids and rutin, and other factors which guard against hemorrhage.

Failing Eyes

Q. *I have had eye trouble and wish to take some carrot juice and would like to know how much to take. Also, is there anything else I could do for this condition?*—A. W., Baxter, Iowa.

A. Carrot juice is good for failing eyes. The dosage is the amount needed to make the changes in the eye symptoms. There are people who have drunk as much as two or three gallons per day. Of course, they eat nothing else. (This makes them turn yellow, which is not a pathological jaundice, so the therapy does not have to be discontinued.)

Another form of treatment is the use of raw, unpasteurized and unfiltered honey. This honey can be put directly into the eye on a daily basis. It stings, so be prepared to suffer for a minute or two. However, there are people who claim to have been cured of eye problems by this simple remedy. Apparently all types of eye problems are helped by honey.

Castor oil applied to the eyes is very soothing and is good for symptomatic relief, but it is not a cure.

Fluorescent Lights

Q. *Several years ago while I was working in the office machine room, an overhead fluorescent lamp burst. Some of the fluorescent dust got into my eyes. After an examination and tests, my eye doctor told me that I have conjunctivitis.*

I am required to wear dark glasses for protection against glare of the sun and am still under the doctor's care. My condition is about the same. Could there be a possible improvement of this condition nutritionally?—Mr. F.P.F., San Diego, California.

A. The treatment, nutritionally, is to give as much support to the local tissue as possible. In this case, the administration of tissue extract of eye* seems to be a must. Naturally, the administration of Vitamins A and C is also a must. In fact, a whole gamut of nutrients is in order.

Eye Muscle Trouble

Q. *I've had an eye muscle problem for about five years that continues to trouble me. I have been to three oculists who tell me there is no disease. Do you have any suggestions?*—N.C.B., Sparta, New Jersey.

A. First, I would institute an exercise program. You should do the child's trick of bringing your finger to your nose from a distance while keeping your finger in focus. This will strengthen the muscles of accommodation. The exercise should be done many times daily, even 100 times twice daily or more. Make your eyeballs accommodate to the finger or pencil. Second, you need hydrochloric acid. Third, you need B complex vitamins and Vitamins A and D.

Eyes Water

Q. *My eyes water very much when I get up in the morning. It continues during the day only not as hard. I am in my 50s and have had it about four years now. The doctors cannot help me. It seems to be worse, especially in the cold weather. Any help you could give me would be greatly appreciated.*—A. M., Milwaukee, Wisconsin.

A. This symptom, like many others, represents the body responding in an insufficient manner because of nutritional deficiencies. First, let me say that insufficiencies develop not only because of insufficient intake, but also because of insufficient digestive capability, poor absorption, inadequate metabolism or too rapid excretion. Any of these can cause imbalances or insufficiencies. This is why it is neces-

*See Product Information.

sary to have a complete metabolic checkup in the first place.

Nearsightedness

Q. *Does a very nearsighted person have to be nightblind?*—E.M., Venango, Nebraska.

A. Nearsightedness is a reaction of the visual apparatus which makes the image fall short of the retina in the eye. This is due in part to the anatomic structure of the eye, but, more importantly, to how the eye functions. There is a gross loss of elasticity so that the eyeball cannot change adequately to accommodate. In part, at least, this can be due to a deficiency of Vitamin A. The function of the eye is closely associated with Vitamin A. Night-blindness is also a sign of deficiency of Vitamin A. Therefore, a nearsighted person stands a good chance of developing nightblindness. Naturally, a completely balanced nutritional diet is basic.

B-Complex Deficiency

Q. *For some reason all the fluid in my mucous membrane seems to be drying up. That goes for my whole body, but I had a severe bout with my right eye last fall. I would try to open my eyes first thing in the morning and they would hurt. They would wake me up in the night, hurting badly. I was almost climbing the walls. Then they would water profusely and would feel better. I would go for about a day without hurting and then start the cycle all over again. One doctor gave me drops for dry eye, another put drops in that would deaden the feeling. I finally went to a specialist and he had to scrape off the skin, or whatever it is over the eyeball, and let new grow. Now the eye is beginning to be hard to open and I have to wink real hard every morning to get it damp enough to open. My eyes are fine all day and the tear ducts function normally. At this point the trouble occurs only in the morning. Do you have any suggestions?*—J.B., Senoia, Ga.

A. Primarily, the problem of dryness of the tissues is

due to a Vitamin-B-complex deficiency. Since the body needs all nutrients in order to be in harmony it is a mat-need sufficient HCl and the digestive enzymes in order to ter of getting the nutrients into the system. Here we also need sufficient HCl and the digestive enzymes in order to get the raw materials into the system to stimulate proper reaction in the different organs.

Eye Hemorrhage

Q. *My right eye hemorrhaged, leaving my vision slightly impaired (small dark spot). Aside from taking large amounts of C complex and bioflavonoid tablets, how can I reduce the likelihood of another hemorrhage? Would following a less tension-filled schedule be of help?*—H. K., Detroit, Michigan.

A. Hemorrhage into the vitreous of the eye is considered a permanent thing. In one instance I accidentally seemed to improve the condition of a patient by using large doses of pantothenic acid. This gentleman had a rather bothersome nasal allergy for which I prescribed 1000 mg of pantothenic acid about six or seven times daily. At first the allergy did not improve but the sight did. Later the allergy did improve—and so did the eyesight. At the start he was hardly able to see my eye chart even at 10 feet with one eye. As time progressed, he was able to see down to the fourth line at 10 feet.

Of course, you need adequate Vitamin E, B complex, calcium and magnesium. In fact, a balanced program including all the necessary nutrients. Bioflavonoids are certainly indicated also.

Eye Hemorrhage

Q. *My husband was examined by an eye doctor and was told that there are some changes in the eyes that make them hemorrhage. He is 77 years old, feels fine, sleeps well and seems to be in fairly good condition. The doctor gave him eye drops—four times a day—sometimes the drops clear his eyes and sometimes they feel inflamed.*

Could you suggest anything that could possibly help the situation?—M.C., Monrovia, California.

A. It is unclear as to whether you are talking about eye hemorrhages in the sclera (the white part of the eye visible on external examination) or whether the hemorrhage is internal, within the eye, and not visible. In either case, the condition seems to be one concerning the capillaries and smaller arterioles and venules. It sounds as if there is a seepage of blood from the capillaries into the tissues, thus being called hemorrhage.

Correction of this condition is found in the approach to strengthening the integrity of the capillaries. First and foremost, is the administration of Vitamin C complex which includes the bioflavonoids. This complex supplies the cementum (collagen) necessary to hold the cellular components together in the capillaries. If the cells are held together, then there is less seepage. The next nutritional item to be considered is calcium. Calcium is necessary for proper coagulation of blood. So is Vitamin K. Vitamin-K deficiency develops when frozen foods are consumed to the exclusion of natural foods. Naturally, a total nutritional program should be in effect in order to correct this condition.

Vitamin K is not available in supplement form but from foods, especially yogurt. It is also found in chlorophyll in precursor form.

Chalazion

Q. *About 10 months ago, I developed four small growths on the lower lid of my left eye. I consulted my family physician who advised that I apply warm compresses and use an ointment he prescribed. After having followed his advice diligently for quite a while these growths still persisted. I decided to go to an eye specialist who informed me that these growths were medically known as multiple chalazions and advised surgical removal. This was accomplished with the exception of one growth which was very close to my tear duct. He said that removal of this particular growth would run the risk of in-*

terfering with tear duct function itself and advised against it. Also, a biopsy was taken and it was found to be non-malignant. I have no pain or discomfort from this growth but it makes me quite self-conscious. I was wondering if you could advise me as to how I might possibly have this removed nonsurgically?—A.Z., Hempstead, N.Y.

A. A chalazion is a glorified abscess of the eyelid which has been present for a long period of time. It tends to become encapsulated so that it recurs at intervals. Medically, the advice was sound in that there is no known method of elimination except by surgical removal.

Nutritionally, there is another approach. This includes the usual anti-infective approach through adequacy of Vitamins A and C in the diet, along with a good balanced and adequate total nutritional approach. I am afraid that this lesion requires something more, however. Since it is a chronic lesion, the infective organism is probably staphylococcus. For this I would use the Staphage Lysate,* SPL. It would be a long term approach of weekly intradermal injections of the SPL. Eventually, the problem would be solved.

There is another approach which I have discovered which is very simple. I use Corona Ointment. This is an animal product used for the treatment of cracks in the nipples of nursing cows. It is an old-time remedy. This ointment is safe to use in the eye. I recommend the application of a good fingerful of the ointment to the eye and rub it in thoroughly. Do this two or three times daily and the lesion may be gone in a few days. I have used this approach personally. This ointment is not considered to be an eye ointment but I have found it to be perfectly safe in a near-the-eye lesion.

Pterygium

Q. *I have what is known as a pterygium in my eye. I've had it for several years during which time I've been told that nothing short of surgical removal can help. Do you have any suggestions?—L.H., Costa Mesa, Ca.*

*See Product Information.

A. A pterygium is a condition on the eyeball where muscles used to move the eye from side to side are enlarged and grow toward the pupil. Sometimes these muscle fibers begin to cover the pupil. Surgical removal is the usual and probably the only sure course. It is possible to take certain nutrients, however, which are favorable to eye metabolism and which could possibly cause the eye to improve. I refer to Vitamins A and D as a starter. Also the B complex and C complex are vital.

Colored Splotches

Q. *I have developed yellowish colored splotches on the whites of my eyes. They are called pingueculas, I believe, by the optometrists. They disturb me as they are so conspicuous, although not painful. Different doctors have different explanations for them—from cholesterol deposits to inflammation caused by weather—but none have remedies. I was wondering if they might not be caused by some nutritional deficiency and could possibly be corrected through sound nutrition? Most doctors don't take that into consideration and I wish you could comment on the problem.*—Mrs. W.R., Eureka, California.

A. You are on the right track. Nutrition can probably do something for you. Unfortunately, there is no easy answer. It is the whole approach that is so important. The weakest areas of the body break down first. Then it spreads to other areas. It may be the same cause, but the reaction may be quite different because of the unique form of the different tissues in the different areas of the body. Your eye problem is a localized reaction to your systemic condition of a disturbance in fat metabolism which can result in the eye spots.

You suggest that this condition could be caused by too much carotene in the diet. I presume you drink carrot juice. It is not the juice that is the primary culprit, but the toxins which have been liberated from the tissues by the juice, and then, while circulating in the blood, have combined with the carotene to cause the yellow discolorations in the tissues. I have not found this effect to be a serious physical problem except from the cosmetic angle. If one just continues to drink carrot juice, the yellowish discolorations will eventually disappear. It could take a long time, but it will happen when the liver is cleansed and the rest of the body reacts accordingly.

Keratoconus

Q. *My son, age 26, has keratoconus. The Air Force found it out in 1967. Now they say in a year he will have to have a cornea transplant. We are very much against this. Will vitamins, zone therapy or any other treatment help his problem? He can see with contacts, but his eyes keep watering and he washes them out.*—Mrs. H.G., Billings, Montana.

A. Keratoconus is a condition of the cornea wherein it protrudes outward in a cone form, like an ice cream cone. There is no known cause mentioned in my reference books. Nutritionally, one may suspect there is some sort of weakness of the cornea which allows this disfiguration to develop. The only nutritional approach which occurs to me is to flood the system with all the nutrients favorable for normal eye function. The total vitamin-mineral intake is basically important. Then there can be stressed certain items like magnesium, Vitamin A in huge doses, Vitamin D, eye tissue extracts and nerve tissue extracts.* I have no proof if this program would be beneficial but it makes sense to assume that it could at least prevent further extension of the problem.

*See Product Information.

18. Female Complaints

Menopause

Q. *I am in my midforties nearing menopause. For the past nine months I have been taking 100 I.U. of Vitamin E daily for leg cramps and cold extremities. The cramps have disappeared and circulation to my extremities has improved, but the broken veins on my legs are becoming very unsightly. I have always had these, but they seem to be getting worse. Could this be a result of the Vitamin E or merely coincidence?*—N. H., Ontario, Canada.

A. You have the correct idea as a start here, but the dosage is insufficient. You must find your own level of Vitamin E by intelligently and deliberately increasing the dosage slowly until the desired results are attained. If you use the mixed tocopherals in the Vitamin E there is less chance of causing an alarming blood pressure increase as can sometimes occur with the d-alpha tocopherol. Providing calcium with enough phosphorus tends to relieve muscle cramps. I stumbled on this answer accidentally. For years I have been using a calcium-magnesium preparation to relieve calcium deficiency symptoms.

I would not hesitate to give you some natural hormones, too. I use the natural estrogen tablets and find that they do much good for female patients. They are not dangerous as the synthetics are.

Estrogens and Menopause

Q. *Can taking estrogen hormones after menopause cause breast cancer and blood clots? A doctor who answers letters in my local newspaper says they can cause blood clots in the menopause woman as well as in young women.*

140

Do you think there is any other natural way a woman can balance out the hormones with Vitamin E and wheat germ oil after menopause?—Mrs. J.H., Gilroy, California.

A. Many women suffer severe torture during and after the menopause. These symptoms, for the most part, can be controlled with estrogens. There are two general divisions of hormones—natural and synthetic—which are available.

Synthetic is made from coal tar sources and, for my money, should not be used because of the possibility of their cancer-causing effect. The natural forms are extracted from pregnant mare urine. This is equestrian estrogen, called *Premarin,* but as far as I know, it is the same as the hormones secreted by human females. I do not hesitate to use this type of hormone except where some sort of cancer already exists in the secondary sex organs such as breasts, uterus, etc., or in the ovaries.

The synthetics on the other hand are used popularly, along with the synthetic progesterone types in the form of the Pill. I consider ALL OF THEM BAD and believe they should not be used under any circumstances if at all avoidable.

There is a natural way to balance out the hormones. This demands, first, an adequate and abundant nutritional balance in the patient. To this is added an eight-to-one concentrate of wheat germ oil. This is known to contain the precursors to the sex hormones and can be utilized by the female. I prefer wheat germ oil perles only because I do not think you can consume the wheat germ oil fast enough to guard against rancidity, which is carcinogenic in itself. Refrigeration only slows down the process of rancidity. The dosage on the perles is variable and must be determined by trial and error. Start with one three times daily and then gradually increase the dosage as need is determined.

Period Problems and Various Complaints

Q. *I am a 17-year-old girl in very bad health, at least I think so. It all started when I went to my family physician for help in ridding myself of broken veins in my legs. (I had had these since I was eight.) He put me on a diet.*

Six months later, I was 25 pounds lighter and I had stopped having my periods and had become constipated. Of course, my family physician said this was "normal" for my age and I would straighten out. We moved to another town and I changed doctors. This doctor also said it was normal.

A while after I started going to this doctor, I began to spit up my food as if it were coming from my esophagus. It was not like vomiting but rather spitting up. The doctor prescribed some medicine (two types) but neither worked. So he suggested that it was my stomach, my gallbladder, my thyroid, or a hiatal hernia. I had blood tests for my thyroid and X rays (G.I. and Gallbladder). My X rays showed nothing and he said my thyroid was "borderline" to hypoactive. He said my stomach problem was probably due to tension and that I would have to learn to control it. (I had been worried and depressed and I would sit and cry for hours.)

Then we made another move—10 miles away. We had been living in our new home for about nine months, and I was still going to the same doctor, and having the same health problems, when he suggested a gynecologist and that I stop all medication. So, I went to the gynecologist. I had not yet had a period for two years, three months. He did a Pap test and could find nothing wrong.

Then I was sent to the lab for another thyroid test and to X ray for skull films for my pituitary gland. He found out my thyroid was past "borderline" and my pituitary was normal. He prescribed progesterone for my periods and synthetic thyroxine for my thyroid. I have had three periods with the progesterone and I am up to taking four, .05 mg, tablets of thyroxine. The gynecologist referred me to an endocrinologist who sent me back to the lab for blood tests for calcium, diabetes and for more X rays of my digestive system. During the X rays, I distinctly heard the doctors say something about a spot on my esophagus. When I returned to the doctor, he said he found nothing in either my blood tests or the X rays.

Every time I call these doctors, they give me a run-around. I know I am ill yet they seem to be doing nothing about it. I have felt bad for almost three years, and I don't think I could stand three more. Do you think that if I went to a doctor who uses no drugs and only natural

*things, he could find out what's wrong with me? I'm really
desperate and about to give up hope.*—Miss J. S., Clemmons, North Carolina.

A. This is a sad but very typical situation which exists
in America today among the orthodox doctors. The name
of the game is to make a diagnosis. If a diagnosis cannot
be made, then there is nothing that can be done for the
patient unless it is a neuropsychiatric sort of treatment.
This is why so many tranquilizers are used. No disease
condition ever develops overnight. There is always a
period during which symptoms gradually become evident
but are not yet well enough organized to point out the diagnosis. The patient is sick but just not sick enough for the
diagnosis to be made. In my experience, the only way to
really know what is happening to a patient is to get as extensive a history as possible; to do a good physical examination, and to do an extensive amount of routine laboratory analyses. Thus, when all this information is assembled
and correlated, the true picture can be ascertained.

My suggestion to you is to get a doctor who will give
you a five-hour seven-specimen glucose tolerance test, and
to be treated for your low blood sugar (which seems a
possibility) and find a good nutritionist to treat you.

Change in Cell Structure

Q. *A recent Pap test at a Los Angeles clinic was compared with the results of the same test taken four years
previously. I was told that a "change in cell structure" was
noted and it was suggested that I return in six months for
another similar test.*

They said no cancer cells were seen.

*Could you tell me what is indicated by a change in
cells? For the past 15 years I've been careful of my food
habits and take many supplements daily. Is there something special I should do in the meantime until the next
Pap test is taken, or just wait to see what it shows?*—F. F.,
Huntington Park, Calif.

A. The Pap test is an examination of the cell structures
seen upon microscopic examination of a certain tissue
scraping. The test was first popularized concerning the

scrapings of the tissues of the female vaginal tract. Later it was found that important information could be obtained by similarly studying other tissue scrapings. In the case of the female vaginal tract, there is a standard classification which is rated as I, II, III, IV. It is generally agreed that a classification of II simply indicates that a recheck should be made after a given period of time. III is a little more definite and does put one into a position of doing something more at the present. This "something more" should consist of a biopsy, according to the accepted medical consensus. One does not go off the "deep end" in regard to the Pap test unless there is confirmatory evidence in some other manner. The case as a whole must be considered.

Personally, I feel that any report other than "I" is indication for action. In classes II and III, I hasten to inaugurate a definite program consisting of basic support, liver detoxification and specific supportive measures. If a definite diagnosis of class IV is made, I immediately refer the patient to another physician for care, even though I will continue to advise her regarding any nutritional problems she may have.

It is my opinion that some of these conditions, before the actual presence of cancer, can be altered so that the inevitable situation does not develop.

Low Estrogen

Q. *My health is very good and I am 50 years old. On my annual physical, my doctor informed me my estrogen is low and explained that if this becomes worse the bones become brittle, etc. He suggested medication either orally or by injection if I agree.*

I have confidence in your opinion and would greatly appreciate a reply on this subject.—F.A., San Francisco, California.

A. It is true that as ovarian function wanes, the bones do become weakened and brittle. The sturdiness of the structure gradually dissolves. One can almost say that this is the normal sequence of events. I say "almost" because I do feel that the osteomalacia and osteoporosis are practically prevented if the diet is strong in the basic nutrients and especially heavy in minerals. First, you need a strong basic nutritional program. You also need a stronger mineral supplementation intake. Finally, the ovaries should be stimulated as much as possible. By this, I mean the added use of raw ovarian tissue extracts.* As a final resort, the use of supplementary hormones comes into the picture. These are substitutive and do tend to suppress normal function of the ovaries. This is an individual matter and must be determined in each individual case.

Amenorrhea

Q. *I am 18, 5'3" and weigh 100 lbs. I have a slight case of acne and I am not very well developed physically. I wear a 32-A bra. I haven't had a period for seven months. I have been irregular for about two years. Before that, I was fine. I tried using Vitamin E—400 units—for a while, but nothing happened. I am concerned that I'll never be normal. Do you have any nutritional advice?—* Miss S.C., Hayward, Calif.

A. You are hypo-ovarian and maybe hypoglandular (hypo means low). You need a complete metabolic evaluation with the development of a strong nutritional program. Orthodoxy can do things with you by the administration of the Pill and other combinations of hormones. Unfortunately, this is not a permanent cure, but one that is maintained only as long as you continue to take the remedy, which I am against.

Pregnancy Drug Reaction

Q. *My O.B. gave me a drug called "Effroxine" during each of my pregnancies for tiredness and morning sickness. I only needed it for the first three months of my first two pregnancies, but relied on it for the whole nine months the last time. He prescribed two tablets a day, each containing five mg. They made me feel like I could*

*See Product Information.

conquer anything while they were working, but when they wore off I became terribly depressed. I couldn't do anything without them. I really became dependent on them. After my third pregnancy, and after the baby was born, I had a nervous breakdown. I fainted easily, crumbled under excitement or strain and became terribly fearful.

I am much better now, the only problems which remain are a periodic anxiety feeling and my eyes are very sensitive to anything, especially light. I lost 15 pounds at the time, which was a lot for me. I weighed 120 and went to 105. I'm 5'4" and my age is 25. It took 18 months to regain my weight and get back on my feet. It's been two years now since my breakdown.

I still can't get anyone to tell me about Effroxine. Many of my friends go to my doctor and are taking this drug. Do you know anything about it? Could you find anything out for me? I would like very much to repair whatever nerve damage may have been done. What can I take that would be a natural healer for this sort of thing? I've been to doctors, internists, neurologists and chiropractors, and all say it's my nerves. That's easy to say, but now what do I do?—Mrs. I.D., West Los Angeles, California.

A. It is not surprising that you have had trouble finding out what is in Effroxine. I could not find the answer in my usual source references. After calling the local druggist, I discovered that this is a methamphetamine, commonly known as "Speed." The drug is on the market under other trade names which I will not mention here. It is a drug controlled under the Class II schedule in the new narcotic law. Your postpregnancy reaction to this drug sounds like hypoglycemia. Hypoglycemia can result after many kinds of stress on the organism which results in an exhaustion of the adrenal cortex glands. In my opinion, this is really a condition of dysnutrition and can be corrected by proper nutritional balance in the system. Help is needed to accomplish this, and the use of adrenocortical extract in large doses is indicated under a definitely controlled plan.

Posthysterectomy Dribbling

Q. *A few years ago I had to have surgery and the uterus was removed. Ever since, I have had trouble holding my water and it's very embarrassing sometimes in a crowd. Is there any exercise I can do or a special vitamin that will help me?*—M.S., Long Beach, California.

A. Posthysterectomy dribbling is a fairly unusual occurrence. This is especially true in the older patient. It is the result of action of the floor of the pelvis where the urethra protrudes from the inner tissues to the outside. Somehow there was damage to the musculature in the floor of the pelvis which prevents the suspension of the urethra in proper manner. I would tend to think that this was not a complication of the surgery, but a complication to the use of a catheter. A catheter left in place too long could weaken the muscles so that they cannot hold the urine. You, in a semiconscious state, could have pulled the catheter from your bladder and, in doing, could have stretched your muscles too much.

Estrogen

Q. *After a hysterectomy I have been taking hormones to control hot flashes. I have been having blood clots about three years now. I have little pain in my legs so I am trying to stay off the estrogen. I am taking 4-5, 200-unit soluble E tablets each day, too. I also take an iron tablet. How long after the iron tablet can I take the estrogen? I hear that they are incompatible.*—M.A., San Jose, California.

A. It is true that these two are incompatible, *if* the iron is inorganic. I do think that iron in a chelated form or in the natural state is not antagonistic to the estrogen or vice versa. However, if there is some doubt in your mind, I would prescribe them to be taken at different times. For instance, take the estrogen at bedtime and the others at breakfast. There is also incompatibility between the estrogen and Vitamin E. Again, the same recommendations.

Hormones

Q. *I have been told that if a person has had a hysterectomy and take the hormone pills, a few years later they won't need them. They could lost their feminine traits—and would become more masculine. Is this true?*—E.J., Petaluma, California.

A. First of all, we must get our terms correct. A hysterectomy is an operation where the uterus has been removed. A total hysterectomy is the same sort of operation only the whole uterus, including the cervix, is removed. Then comes the pan-total hysterectomy. In this operation, the uterus, cervix and the ovaries and tubes are all removed.

If the ovaries are not removed, there continues to be the normal production of estrogen and other female hormones. In other words, there is no need for hormone therapy unless the need already existed or develops as a normal sequence of age.

In this case, I assume you are talking about the condition where the ovaries have been removed. The age of the patient makes a great deal of difference where the determination of hormone substitution is concerned. The younger the patient, the more urgent the substitution. This is so because there is more hormonal shock in the younger woman than in the older woman who is already declining in the hormone production in her system. Thus you can see that substitutional therapy is controlled to a certain extent by the age of the patient. Age also influences the duration of therapy. The treated patient can take hormones for a considerable length of time and then there can be a "normal" withdrawal corresponding to the menopause and postmenopause periods of time. If one wishes to become extreme, as some are doing today, the therapy can be continued on and on, well into the 70s and 80s; even to the point of having regular periods. To each her own. I prefer to gradually reduce the dosage so that the decline in the later years is lessened, but I do not go along with the maintenance of the cycle much longer than it normally would continue.

Another point to remember is that when the ovaries are removed, the adrenal glands then become the prime producers of estrogens and female hormones as well as the male hormones, in the female. Each of us produces a combination of both types of hormones.

Now for the patient in question: I would give her hormone therapy so that the sudden removal of the major hormone production centers would not create a crisis in her life. There would have to be a maximum amount of hormone dosage in this case. Gradually, as the menopause years are past and she is well into the postmenopause period, the dosage can be reduced. To a certain extent, there can be a masculinization of the characteristics because male hormones are still being produced by the adrenals. But in general, this amount of masculinization would only be the amount or about the amount that would have been expected even if there had been no surgery.

Just a word about the types of hormones to be used. I am a firm believer that the synthetic hormones *should not be used* because of possible carcinogenic activity. I do not feel that this danger is present in the use of the natural hormones, called natural conjugated estrogens, usually derived from pregnant mare urine. I consider this safe for extended use. I am definitely against the Pill which is a synthetic combination of estrogen and progesterone or similarly derived formulations. The Pill is a danger to everyone who takes it—all you have to hear is what doctors' malpractice insurance companies say about it and you will be convinced.

Hysterectomy

Q. *I am 26 and a year ago I had a complete hysterectomy. Now I am taking large doses of estrogen (250 mg daily). I asked my doctor what would happen if I didn't take them and he said I'd get hot flashes and dizzy spells. I recently read where estrogen produces cancer in rats and am wondering about continuing the use of this medicine. I've also read where Vitamin E can take care of hot flashes and dizziness. Can you help?*—S.M., Chillicothe, Ohio.

A. Without the ovaries, you are headed almost instantly into the menopause and all its grueling experiences, hot flashes and all. You are indeed lucky if the doctors have been able to control your problem with hormones. I do hope they are natural hormones so that you, at least, avoid the great cancer exposure that the synthetics cause. You certainly can do something helpful by using large dosages of Vitamin E. Remember that the E must be taken at a time eight to twelve hours away from the hormones or else one may neutralize the other.

Endometriosis

Q. *I have a serious question to ask you. My daughter has a condition called Endometriosis. So far the only solution offered is complete removal of the female organs including the ovaries. Would you be kind enough to tell me if, as far as you know, this is the only solution for such a condition?*—M.B., Los Angeles, Ca.

A. Endometriosis is a condition of the female during the menses when there is a backflow of the menstrual material up into the tubes and thence into the peritoneal cavity. This material eventually becomes implanted into the various intraperitoneal organs and structures so that there are small colonies of endometrial tissue growing in an abnormal place. Then, when the hormonal control comes along to cause the regular menstrual pattern, this implanted tissue goes through all the same changes as does the normal tissue located within the uterus. Each of these little implants has its own period.

This condition is a real problem to those who suffer from it. There are a couple of nutritional steps which should be tried before such drastic measures as surgery are undertaken.

The first is to establish a good basic supplementation program to be sure that there is an adequacy of all the vitamins, minerals, proteins, fats and carbohydrates. Once established one can become more concerned about the specific environment of the organs in question. Vitamin E has a lot to do with normal ovarian action and should be used in adequate dosages. One should also give the raw tissue extracts* of both the ovaries and uterus a chance. One should thoroughly check out the thyroid to verify normal action of this gland. A deficiency of calcium could have been the original problem. It works like this: deficiencies of calcium can and do cause spasms of muscles. The cervix is a very strong muscular-sphincter type structure. Shortages of calcium could cause spasms of this muscle in the crucial time of the menses so that the flow cannot be eliminated. Since it must go some place, it goes up the tubes into the peritoneal cavity.

Solving the calcium problem is not always easy. It must be in adequate supply in the diet. It must be balanced with magnesium, sodium, potassium and other trace minerals, Vitamin D and parathyroid hormone. Acid is also needed for its assimilation.

Cervix Problems

Q. For several years, I have been involved with doctors who recommend pills, cauteries, cryotherapy treatments—you name it, because I have a "spot" on the mouth of my womb. The doctor cannot give me a name for it. He says it appears to the eye as a brushburn on the arm. I went to one doctor for two years and he kept telling me—"It's almost gone. Just use this one more tube of cream and that should do it." Not knowing that it could become "serious" (as he said: "it's minor"), I believed him. Well it has never "quite gone." Finally, I went through surgery for two cysts on my ovary adhesions, and my appendix was removed. The womb was left alone. Now, only nine months later, I am told that the handwriting is on the wall—and within one year to 18 months, the womb must go. I have no children.

They speak of surgery as something that you get over in three days. I am not afraid of the thought of surgery—that is not what is bothering me. But, two operations within that short a time—being cut on the same place twice—

*See Product Information.

is asking a lot. Could you please give me any nutritional advice you know that would solve this problem?—B.R., Metairie, Louisiana.

A. First, one must be sure that all the basic nutritional elements are included in the diet abundantly. Not only should you eat as much fresh, raw items as possible, but you should also supplement the intake with abundant amounts of all the nutrients. Large doses of Vitamin A are very healing for skin and mucous membrane. Vitamin C helps to increase resistance wherever help like this is needed in the body. Maybe larger doses of Vitamin E would be worth a trial. I cannot guesstimate your needs without a complete metabolic examination. Even then it is difficult to determine with certainty.

One of the greatest dangers of having two surgeries is the effect of anesthetics. Double exposure to fluorine-type anesthetics can cause liver damage, even to a fatal degree. Don't let anyone tell you that anesthetic drugs are not potentially dangerous.

Fibroid Tumors

Q. *I am concerned for my sister who has fibroid tumors. One location is the uterus and presently it makes the uterus appear to be the size of an 18- to 20-week pregnancy. She has had these for three years and was told she could not get pregnant and was taken off the Pill whereby she became pregnant. She was told by her physician that she would be lucky to carry this baby. In fact, in his 25 years of practice, only twice (and hers being the second) had any of his patients become pregnant with such tumors. She carried the child the full nine months and both mother and child appear to be very healthy. Her doctor wants to do a hysterectomy (removing the uterus, cervix, and if need be, the ovaries, and if necessary—then the Fallopian tubes). She is only 34 and has one child.*

While I was home visiting, I suggested and arranged an appointment at a university hospital for a staff doctor to examine her. He feels the first doctor's judgment was correct and that leaving the tumors there and growing (she has been back on the Pill—doesn't it cause tumors to grow?) could cause damage to ovaries and then she would go through the complete change.

I was told by a nutritionist that chlorophyll, two tablets in a half-pint of water per douche per day plus 900 units of Vitamin E will reduce the tumor size. Is this true? Are you aware of any measure other than surgery?—J.C., Oakland, California.

A. The only reasons for performing hysterectomies for fibroids are: infection, bleeding and excessive size. In this case, we have a normally functioning uterus which contains fibroids. To do or not to do a hysterectomy is the question. Frankly, the reasons for performing such an operation do not fulfill the above-mentioned criteria. It would be interesting to know how the doctor justifies his recommendation for surgery.

You suggest a chlorophyll douche to reduce the size of the tumor along with Vitamin E. I do not know that either will accomplish the job.

Fibroid Tumor

Q. *I am 44 years old, single, slim, 5' 6½" weigh 130, with no children. Five months ago I found out I have a fibroid tumor in my uterus. The doctor told me it was about the size of an egg. Five months later, when Dr. Shute checked me, he said it was about the size of a 3½-month pregnancy. I also have Raynaud's syndrome. What can be done nutritionally for these problems?*—S. M., Pontiac, Michigan.

A. A fibroid tumor is a muscular type growth within the myometrium or muscular layer of the uterus. It tends just to get larger without growing. It is the result of imbalance of the female hormones, especially the lack of progesterone. Injections of progesterone on a weekly basis for a while will help to rid your body of the tumor. This must be injected because, to the best of my knowledge, it is destroyed by the stomach juices when taken by mouth.

In regard to supplements for fibroids, I have little to offer. The use of agents to normalize the function of the ovaries is important. I use raw ovarian tissue extract for this purpose. It does help to a certain degree. I also use Vitamin E and wheat germ oil concentrates by mouth in an attempt to normalize the function of the ovaries.

Vaginal Infection

Q. *About a year ago I went to a doctor because of a vaginal infection. (I was 21, it was my first such infection.) He explained to me that it was a contamination from the rectum and that my husband acquired the same infection through sexual intercourse and harbored it in his prostate. Therefore he treated both of us to prevent reinfection. We took the drugs and I had no more trouble. Yet recently I developed a vaginal infection with the same itching and general irritation. Similarly, my husband complained of a more-frequent-than-usual, extremely urgent need to urinate. We are wondering if this can be a symptom of harboring such an infection in his prostate, and if there is any nutritional approach we can use to clear up this infection.*—C.Z., Parma, Ohio.

A. It certainly does sound as if you are suffering from a repeat performance. It is quite apparent that you harbored the infection only to have it crop out again at this time. Nutritionally, you must aim at a complete body program. There is nothing special except for the use of large doses of Vitamins A and C.

However, there is a very good method of treatment for this case which is about as natural as possible under the circumstances. I would use Staphage Lysate.* This substance can be used to cause the body to increase its resistance toward staphylococcus to such an extent that there may be a spillover of resistance toward other bodily threats. Your infection by now is probably a mixed type of infection and more than likely does contain some staph. You should benefit by this approach. The dosage I would probably use under these circumstances would be 0.1cc. intradermally—weekly for at least twelve weeks. In all probability, I would use it for much more than the twelve weeks to be sure that the body had built up adequate de-

*See Product Information.

fense against this type of infection. One can expect a reaction around the site of the injection. It can be small like a dime or it can be several inches in diameter. There can even be a systemic reaction sometimes with a fever and malaise for a day or so. In the great majority of cases, the reaction is tolerable and the patient has no real problems so long as he looks forward to the final, good results.

Vaginal Infection

Q. *A recent Pap test revealed I have pus cells in my urine. I also have low grade infection in my vagina. The doctor gave me an injection (I neglected to ask what it contained) and a prescription for Prostaphlin. I don't like taking drugs or medication of any kind. Is there any way this condition can be cleared up by natural methods without resorting to medication?*—E.B., Milwaukee, Wis.

A. Pus cells in the vaginal tract can be brought under control by douching. I use different types such as: apple cider vinegar, using two tablespoonfuls to one quart of warm water. Use as a douche twice daily. One can also use a douche of Golden Seal. Another is to make a solution of sea salt—one teaspoonful per quart warm water and add one tablespoonful of three percent hydrogen peroxide. Use this douche twice daily.

Vaginal Infection

Q. *Could you please tell me the nature of monilia albicans, the duration of it, and what method or natural treatment there is to combat it or counteract it?*—C.B., Ashford, West Virginia.

A. Monilia albicans is a yeast and tends to invade the vaginal area after antibiotic therapy. The complication of having monilia albicans after antibiotic therapy is a real problem. Fortunately, it does not happen often. My personal form of treatment is the use of a 10 percent solution of gentian violet, plus five percent acriflavin in glycerine. I use this by application into the vaginal vault on a weekly basis until the infestation is eradicated. It usually does not take very many treatments. It is also very messy.

Trichomonas Vaginitis

Q. *Would you please give me any information possible on the female disorder, trichomonas? I have had this for the past three months and can't seem to get rid of it. The doctor has had me on drugs two different times, but as soon as I quit taking them it comes back. I don't like taking drugs of any kind. Is there some nutritional way of taking care of this problem? Is there something that my husband or I might do to alleviate it?—Mrs. D.W., Reno, Nevada.*

A. Trichomonas vaginitis is a one-celled animal or protozoa commonly located in the intestinal tract but mislocated into the vaginal tract. It causes a local reaction with inflammation and production of a vaginal discharge. It is difficult to control once it gets established. It does cause the normal acidity of the vaginal mucosal discharge to become alkaline so this gives us the first clue for treatment: get the acidity back to the vaginal tract; then do something to eliminate the organism from the area. My method is to have the patient douche with an apple cider vinegar twice daily for the first week and once daily for the next two weeks. The proportions here are: 2 tbsp. of apple cider vinegar (not distilled vinegar) to one quart of warm water. After the douching, I suggest the insertion of an herb, Gold Seal, tablet into the vaginal tract. Leave the tablet in place until the next douche. A three-week course like this usually clears up the infestation.

Vaginal Discharge

Q. *For the past month or so, I have been fighting a vaginal discharge that is abnormal At first, it was a white discharge, but sometimes seems to be of a gelatinous nature and yet, again, it is quite watery. I am 48 years old, but do not think I am going through the menopause,* *although my periods have lessened from about five days to about two days. There is sometimes a burning sensation around the vaginal opening but no itchiness. A vinegar douche relieves it but it always returns a day or so later. Do you have any suggestions?—H. A., Santa Rosa, Cal.*

A. I gather that there does not seem to be any infection present which would produce pus in the discharge. A discharge of this type is not particularly associated with the menopause which you could be entering at this age of 48. However, it is not unusual to have a discharge at this period of life. After you have been examined to eliminate any sort of serious pathology, the first attempt should be Vitamin E. Choose a good mixed tocopherol type preparation and take 100 I.U. to start. In about a month, if there is no improvement, try a larger dosage. I would keep on increasing the dosage up to maybe 1,000 to 1,500 I.U. per day. The next step would be to take a 1:8 concentration of wheat germ oil.* Take up to two, three times daily. Raw ovarian tissue extract could be an answer, too. This substance increases the action of the ovary, and tends to rejuvenate the gland. Finally, if all else fails, one could use *natural* estrogen supplementation such as Premarin. This is not the same as the synthetic varieties and does not cause the complications.

Hygiene Sprays

Q. *My teenage daughter has had an odor from the vaginal area for many years and so far as we know, not from any discharge, as our doctor is unable to find anything wrong. Is there anything that could be done to eliminate this odor as, needless to say, it's quite embarrassing for her. She had been using these feminine hygiene sprays— but now we are concerned for we've read and heard that these products have been causing injury to people because of the ingredients they contain. What could she use that would eliminate this odor and yet be safe?—Mrs. E.B., Des Plaines, Illinois.*

A. The simplest thing that I can think of to attempt to

*See Product Information.

remedy this condition is to use a douche consisting of apple cider vinegar and sea salt. The ratio is two tablespoonfuls of vinegar, two teaspoonfuls of salt and one quart of warm water. This should be used twice daily until results are forthcoming. Then it can be cut to a bedtime usage. Later it can be gradually phased out as she demonstrates that less intensive therapy is needed.

Another approach would be large oral dosages of Vitamin C. Here, the dosage should be in the range of 20,000–30,000 mg per day. I have not tried using Vitamin C douches with my patients, but a three percent solution of ascorbic acid could be used as a douche without harm.

If these simpler methods do not bring response in the patient, she should have a complete metabolic evaluation. Actually, this condition probably represents some sort of abnormal metabolic response.

CYSTS

Q. *My problem is cysts or cystic mastitis of the breasts. Every six months I have a checkup and find cysts. I can find no answer to prevent this condition. Can you help me?*—Mrs. M.T., Tucson, Arizona.

A. Orthodoxy cannot tell the difference between a benign cyst and a malignant tumor without biopsy. Eventually, you will be persuaded to have both breasts amputated so that this problem will no longer exist.

Nutritionally, I can be of little help. I once read that high doses of Vitamin A would correct cystic diseases. You would probably need upward to 100,000 I.U. or more each day. Contrary to FDA accusations, this is not a toxic dosage to the overwhelming majority of individuals—only to a few people. It is also possible that stimulation of pituitary and thyroid to midnormal function would be of some value. Thyroid can be normalized by use of iodine, pituitary by use of raw pituitary extract. It is also possible that the pituitary function can be influenced by bromide since this is the concentration location for the body.

Cystocele or Rectocele

Q. *I am a longtime subscriber to the belief in natural health. I do not want to have to be checked by a doctor and then be obliged to take his antibiotics and whatever else, but I must do something. What methods and what possible exercises could I follow to overcome a large bulge in my vagina?*— V.F., Yucaipa, Calif.

A. You probably have either a cystocele or rectocele, or both. These conditions are dependent upon what part of the abdominal contents are forcing themselves outward through the vagina. Both conditions represent a weakness of the muscular and fibrous tissue formation of the floor of the true pelvis. At this point, the tissues are acting like a rubber band that has been spent. What you can do nutritionally is minimal at best. Once damage is done, there is little to be done to recover normalcy of tissues. I would try large mineral dosages, particularly manganese.

Ovarian Cyst

Q. *I have been told that I have a cyst on my left ovary. Is there any way to get rid of this cyst other than by surgery?*—T.S., Golden, Colorado.

A. Ovarian cysts are a peculiar problem. Cysts are perfectly normal. One matures and ruptures every time you have a period. It subsides immediately after the period. If pregnancy ensues, then the cyst shell develops into the corpus luteum. This is a vital structure in the pregnancy period. The so-called cyst which needs to be removed surgically may be one of those types of cysts that have matured improperly or have not disappeared. They could also be malignant, though this is not so common.

The total nutritional program should be adopted with special reference to Vitamin E and ovarian cytotrophic products. The latter should be started slowly with an enzymatic extract of ovarian tissue.* One could conceivably cause the cyst to grow excessively or to cause hemorrhage.

*See Product Information.

Both of these complications should be avoidable by slowly instituting the dosage necessary. It is very difficult to accomplish this so it is quite possible that, since you already have a cyst, it will have to be removed surgically. There is a big difference between getting something to go away and preventing it in the first place.

Ovarian Cyst

Q. *Has there been any reported research of successful treatment of an ovarian cyst other than surgery?*—Mrs. I.M.M., Arlington, Virginia.

A. Taking preventive measures before a condition develops is quite successful as compared to what can be done after the condition does develop. If you wish to do something other than surgery, try taking an appropriate dosage of Vitamin E. You should also have all the minerals and vitamins in abundance. Raw ovarian tissue extract* should also be used. I certainly do not hold out any substantial hope, but it is certainly worth a try.

Sterilization

Q. *Do you know of any harmful side effects resulting from sterilization of women by means of tying the tubes? Would such an operation have long-range effects on the heart or nervous system, or result in accelerated aging? Could it bring on premature menopause? Would there be any hormone disturbance?*—Mrs. R. C., Haverford, Pennsylvania.

A. Sterilization of women by the ligation of the tubes is quite a common procedure. It is almost without complication but is not commonly done as a primary procedure. In other words, the procedure is done in conjunction with some other surgery, but not as a primary reason for surgery. It is a very simple procedure. The tubes are simply tied in the midportion by a ligature that is looped around the tube and tightened. Some surgeons get carried away

*See Product Information.

and tie in two places and then excise the tube between. Oddly enough, they then tie the two loose ends of the tube close together, theoretically to guarantee the closing of the tubes by scar tissue. This is always done on both tubes.

The result of this procedure is simply to prevent the ovum from going down the tube from the ovary to the uterus. It also prevents the sperm from ascending up into the tube where fertilization usually takes place. The woman still has her usual periods with absolutely no obvious alteration. There is no difference in the hormonal production of the ovaries. The blood supply to the ovaries is not altered at all so the distribution of hormones is absolutely unaltered. Since the hormones are not changed, then there is no effect on the aging process. Thus, also, the bringing on of premature menopause is not to be a part of this procedure at all. There is no disturbance in the physiology of the person except the egg and the sperm do not have a chance to come in contact.

Bust Size

Q. *I have a problem which may seem minor to you but to me it is quite a disappointment. Seven years ago when I got married my bust measurement was a pleasant 36-A and now after three babies I am down to 32½ inches around the bust even though I have gained 10 pounds otherwise. I have tried all kinds of exercises for this and nothing seems to help. Is there any way of getting the proper hormone through eating?*—L.D., Scott City, Kansas.

A. I would assume from your brief letter that your bust measurement in the prechild state was due to fat deposits in the breast. Now they are more glandular in nature. Since the glands are only maximally active while pregnant and nursing, the lessened size is due to the alteration in physical size of the glands. I know of no way to cause fat to be redeposited into the breast mass to cause an enlargement.

I hear there are breast exercisers on the market worth a try.

Flat Breasts

Q. *Since weaning my baby my breasts have been flat and shapeless. Can nutrition be of any help?*—S. G. F., Daytona Beach, Florida.

A. This is a common occurrence. Where tissues are used to the maximum and then not used to the maximum, there can be and usually is a sagging result. There just is not the amount of underlying structures to maintain the normal shape. To a certain extent, one can guard against such a reaction by adequate stimulation through exercise and massage.

In spite of the good care for breasts in the postlactation period, breasts just sag after lactation. Vitamin E, a B complex and lecithin may help.

Certain exercises, like the push-type—palms of hands against each other—have helped some people.

Bust Development

Q. *I have tried my best to increase my bustline with weight lifting and exercise. I have successfully firmed my pectoral muscles, but that seems to be all. I work out regularly and practice health improvements such as saunas, swimming daily, and drinking a pint to a quart of carrot juice every other day. I am interested not only in my bodily appearance, but important organ functioning as well.*—Mrs. J. C., San Antonio, Texas.

A. First, some basics. You are what you are because of age, sex, occupation, place of residence, nutritional pattern, past history, heredity, etc. You are what you are because of all the things which have ever happened to you to make you what you are. Heredity is important. Just look at your mother. If she is small-breasted, you are likely to be.

What can be done? You have already said that you eat well and take exercises and vitamins. You might add raw mammary tissue extract* to your intake. There are some cases where this has aided in expanding the bust line.

*See Product Information.

Facial Hair

Q. *I know a young girl, aged 32, who has such a strong growth of hair on her chin that it resembles men's whiskers. As a result she feels it necessary to shave daily. My question is this: is there any natural way to stimulate her hormone balance and thus stop this growth which is so unusual on young women?*—J. W., Hudson, N.H.

A. Increased facial hair in females is not as rare as you seem to imply. The cause, in my estimation, is failure of the female sex glands, and excessive function of adrenal cortices. Things such as Vitamin E and a general nutritional program are helpful in correcting this problem. It is also wise to stimulate the ovaries to do their work more perfectly. This can be done by the use of raw ovarian tissue extract.*

However, many cases do not respond to the therapy. Then we have to examine the function of the adrenal glands, particularly the cortices. Sometimes an error of metabolism can be found here. Further investigation brings in the pituitary gland as well as thyroid. It is not an easy problem to solve and many times it seems to evade a solution.

Hair Growth

Q. *My wife, age 47, and now my daughter, age 17, have tremendous growth of hair over most of their skin area. What natural or organic substance may be taken either to arrest or eliminate this condition?*—B.C., Philadelphia, Pennsylvania.

A. This growth of hair is quite unusual. You do not mention if it is distributed in specific areas or if it is just generalized all over. I presume it is masculinizing in nature. The usual answer is that it is hormonal. There is a definite lack of the female hormone and an overabundance of the male hormone. In the female, this usually also means an overactivity of the adrenal cortex glands. This

*See Product Information.

could be in the form of a tumor, either benign or malignant. It could also be an overaction of the pituitary gland which would, in turn, stimulate the adrenal cortices. Since you mention the presence of this condition in both your daughter and wife, I assume that there is some sort of family problem here. It could even be due to a thyroid deficiency.

It is necessary to get a hormone analysis to measure the activity of the various glands which may be involved. This is too complex a subject to go into here, but some answers could be forthcoming from such studies.

Aftereffects of the Pill

Q. *Ever since I started taking the Pill about seven years ago, I have had a vaginal discharge. It started with a discharge with itching, and the itching was cleared up with an antibiotic suppository. The discharge, however, has persisted even though I have been off the Pill over two years now. Also, I have none of the normal secretions to facilitate intercourse.*—Y.S., Atlanta, Georgia.

A. One of my antisubjects is the Pill! This is one of the worst evils I have ever seen propagandized onto the public. The only one which is worse, in my estimation, is the great fluoridation hoax. The Pill can do so many abnormal things to women that I will not even begin to list them. One side effect is in the form of unusual vaginal discharge. Naturally, the treatment is to use antibiotics. So you have now "solved" the discharge problem but have another one in its place. As we all know, antibiotics kill the bacteria indiscriminately—good as well as the bad ones. Thus, the vagina has been left with an abnormal bacterial flora which is not conducive to the normal secretion during intercourse.

How to overcome this is the name of the game. It is not easy many times, though it may be a simple answer sometimes. By putting a culture of friendly bacteria into the vagina one can overcome the bad bacteria. The normal pH of the vaginal secretion is slightly acid. Logically, then, the first thing to do is to try to make the vaginal secretion acid. Check with litmus paper to see if you are alkaline or acid. If alkaline, you should begin to douche with vinegar.

While in medical school, I was told to use this, but not told that the vinegar needed to be apple cider vinegar and not distilled. Since I was trained to think in terms of "purity," I told patients to use the distilled vinegar. It did not work and so I discarded this as being just a joke, until I learned some of the differences between distilled and apple cider vinegars. I found that the latter worked in douches where the former did not. First, then, you should douche *twice daily with a good apple cider vinegar mixture in the* ratio of two tablespoonsful in a quart of warm water. Simply changing the pH of the vaginal secretion makes it very difficult for abnormal bacteria to live there. Thus the area is cleaned. You may not have the right bacteria present yet, but at least the bad ones are fading out.

Next, one can instill cultures of acidophilus bacteria. Use a douching technique. There are several good preparations available in the health food stores as well as drug stores, which can be used. It can be instilled simply by taking the capsule apart and then inserting the contents. This can be done after each douching. Acidophilus yeast can also be used here. It is a little sturdier and can become implanted a little easier. This yeast, as the name implies, is very friendly with the associated bacteria.

Finally, it may be necessary for a doctor to administer hormones to perpetuate the influence of said hormones on the vaginal mucosa and its secretions.

The Pill and Thyroid Problems

Q. *I would like to know what birth control pill you recommend as the safest, healthwise, and do I need more vitamins when on the pill?*

Also I have an underactive thyroid, resulting from a thyroidectomy due to an overactive thyroid. I am taking three grains per day of a substitute thyroid hormone. Do I need any special vitamins for this problem?—H.L.G., Hillside, New Jersey.

A. Birth control pills are an anathema to me. I do not know of any excuse for using them. They are dangerous and contribute to many health problems in women who indulge in them. Just the other day I was fortunate in getting a newly married woman to stop taking them. She came to me for the first time two weeks after her marriage, complaining of severe lower abdominal pains of a few days' duration. On examination, it was rather obvious that there was marked congestion of the veins around the ovaries and that this, to me, was a danger area. With proper treatment, she subsided very nicely and decided not to take the Pill anymore. Is your health worth this kind of gamble? Just use a diaphragm and jelly or foam. If you insist on taking the Pill, please take extra B complex, especially B-6.

Your thyroid problem is a rather common one. Just because you are living on substitute thyroid hormones does not mean that you do not also need a complete nutritional intake. In specific terms, you do need iodine. One source of this mineral is from the sea. I use a preparation of sea sponge, but kelp is also a good source of this mineral. One can get too much iodine but it is fairly hard to do so when taken in this natural form. Better yet, take one drop daily of half strength (½ iodine, ½ water) tincture of iodine.

More About The Pill

Q. *For three years I took birth control pills. Four months ago I stopped and my complexion is breaking out. Most of these lumps are underneath the surface and usually stay two to three weeks. This is very depressing, especially since I care a lot about my appearance. I am wondering if there is something I can do to help keep my face clear once and for all. I read that the Pill depletes the body of Vitamin E. Is this true? Does it rob the body of other nutrients? How can I get myself in proper condition now that I'm off the Pill? Can you help me?*—Mrs. S.J., St. Petersburg, Florida.

A. It sounds as if your acne is the result of having taken the Pill. This is not an unusual complaint. It does tell me from the nutritional aspect, that the Pill has caused an insult to the kidneys. When the skin breaks out, it means to me that there is an overload on the kidneys, thus you need support for the kidneys. In my experience, the use of the raw kidney tissue extract is indicated.* Another tablet is the one consisting of an enzymatic extract of rice polish and beet leaves. It acts as a kidney cleanser.*

It is difficult to state where the action of the Pill is in the nutritional picture. It does detract from the nutritional picture somewhere. I would suggest you have a complete metabolic examination wherein the deficiencies in your own body are detected. Your reaction to the Pill is individual. Naturally, a full complement of all the basic nutrients is in order. I would suspect a defect in the sugar tolerance curve at this point. The Pill contains hormones which do destroy Vitamin E if taken together. Taking both substances 12 hours apart prevents this loss. The Pill also wastes B-6 from your system.

The Pill

Q. *I am 22 years old and have had a problem with my menstrual cycle for about a year. I started taking birth control pills when I was 17 and discontinued them because I was no longer having a menstrual period. My gynecologist first told me to wait a few months and my cycle should return to normal. When this did not happen, I received hormones and various blood and urine tests followed. I was found to be deficient in the pituitary hormone FSH and informed that nothing could be done to correct the situation. I was told that there was no harm in not menstruating and that if I wanted to become pregnant, they could give me a hormone to cause ovulation. My first question is to find out if it is true that no harm is done and if maybe there is a way to correct this.*

Secondly, since discontinuing the birth control pills, my skin has become very badly blemished with acne, though it was clear when I took the Pill. I questioned my doctor, who informed me that since I was not ovulating, I was not producing progesterone and the deficiency of it most likely caused my bad skin condition. I have tried every nutritional and herbal remedy I know of to help my skin but it has been of no avail. I have been an ovo-lacto-vegetarian

*See Product Information.

*for eight months and I eat only natural, unrefined foods.
In addition to a balanced diet I take brewer's yeast,
lecithin, kelp, B-12, wheat germ, Vitamins A and E daily.
I also get plenty of fresh air, sunshine, exercise, and practice yoga regularly. But still my skin problem persists. I
would greatly appreciate any comments, opinions or references that would shed some light on my problem.—J.L.R.,
Roseville, California.*

A. The Pill, which is strong enough to control menstrua-
tion and pregnancy, is certainly strong enough to do other
things in the body. You are reaping the "benefits" of some
of these actions. You certainly do have ovarian deficiency,
probably adrenal, thyroid and pituitary deficiencies, also.
You need a complete metabolic evaluation and therapeutic
program which should include tissue supplementation with
the particular glandular substances involved.

Your diet may be a point of difficulty, too, because it is
hard to get enough protein and B-12 in a lacto-vegetarian
diet. You must work on it as a project. If you do this, then
the diet is quite satisfactory. Do not think you are safe just
because you do not eat meat.

The Pill

Q. *I've read that birth control pills cause deficiencies of
B-6, folic acid and zinc. In your research have you found
other deficiencies caused by the Pill? I've suddenly developed anemia. Complete blood tests have not returned
but I've never had anything close to anemia before and
am very surprised as I take protein, Vitamins A and D,
brewer's yeast, liver pills, wheat germ, lecithin, E, bone
meal, dolomite, kelp, enzymes, C and bioflavonoids. I feel
birth control pills caused this anemia. Have you found any
such study to support this idea?—Mrs. M.J.D., Woodbridge,
Va.*

A. You have answered your own question. Folic acid is
essential for the prevention of anemia. Since the Pill does
interfere with folic acid activity, then a certain number of
women taking the Pill will become anemic as a result.

Folic acid in 5 mg size is not available to anyone,

even to the doctors for prescription purposes, due to FDA interference and desire for control of vitamins.

The FDA is trying to also control Vitamin E, and is already controlling A and D. I suggest you either give up the Pill or take more brewer's yeast to supply folic acid, or both.

19. Foods

Historical Notes

Q. *I was wondering about the 1800s when only natural foods were used, unsprayed, etc.—sound nutrition—how come there was diphtheria, fever-caused illness, etc?*—C. S., New York, New York.

A. A century ago, generally speaking, these diseases existed because of the marked lack in sanitary controls. The disposal of wastes was not controlled so that there was contamination of foods. Before antisepsis, the surgeons did not even wash hands before going into the surgical room. These diseases you mention mostly occurred in populated centers where cross-contamination of the food supply did exist.

Another point to remember is that the diet was not all natural and organic. Sugar was already a problem. So was white flour. One could also speculate regarding the possibility that the diets were not balanced. Even then, when everything was cheap, all the people did not eat balanced diets. In fact, the rich, as today, who could afford the delicacies and did not eat the basics, did suffer from malnutrition.

Blood Sugar

Q. *In a recent physical examination, a fairly high level of sugar was found in my blood. My food is practically devoid of sugar and I take many natural vitamin supplements. Could you please tell me if sugar is used in vitamin tablets and capsules? Thank you.*—Mrs. B.K., Brooklyn, New York.

A. Sugar is used in many preparations. It is found in capsup, in hot dogs, in sugar-coated pills—even some vitamin tablets—in all sorts of canned foods and elsewhere. Let us assume that it is present, until proven otherwise. I do not know the brands of vitamins you use, but there could be sugar in them. Read labels. You are your own detective.

White sugar is a highly processed "foodless" food. All its natural associated factors are removed. It is chemically "pure" and comes as close to being only pure calories as anything I know. For metabolism of sugar within the body, the Vitamin B complex is necessary. All its own supply of Vitamin B has been refined out of sugar cane in making white sugar, so the body must rob other sources of B complex to metabolize white sugar, which causes B deficiencies elsewhere.

Sugar seems to have priority in the body's use of B factors, so that it is capable of robbing body tissues and creating shortages of vitamins. The results are variable, depending upon which tissue has been robbed. As a result, nerve tissue begins to work abnormally. This is evidenced by pain in various nerve areas, such as in the hands or feet. This is called neuritis, or polyneuritis if it occurs in various areas at the same time. Very commonly, it affects the nerves to the heart, and then we have a disturbance in the function of the heart which could result in a heart attack. Coronary heart disease has even been called American beriberi. If acute deficiency develops in the gastrointestinal tissue, which is another common site of Vitamin-B deficiency symptoms, one gets colitis.

Since there is no known cause for cancer, one cannot say that anything, including sugar, is a causative element. I *can* say emphatically, however, that white sugar does not do one single thing to protect the body from cancer. Protection is important. Since we do not know the cause of cancer, the only logical thing to do is to try to build up our general resistance as much as possible.

Animal Protein

Q. *Do you believe that animal protein is safe to eat? Is it advisable in the case of a fibroid tumor, and if not, is this diet I have included adequate, or how could it be im-*

proved upon? The area where I live is bereft of any great interest in nutrition, so I feel somewhat stranded, and don't know quite where to seek advice.—D.M., Muncie, Indiana.

A. Animal protein is safe to eat. It is the additives and contaminants which are unsafe. All you need is digestive capability in order to get proper nourishment from meat. This means plenty of hydrochloric acid in the stomach; lots of bile in the liver secretion and plenty of good pancreatic juice. If you are blessed with these, you can eat almost anything natural and do well. If you do not have the digestive capability, then you are getting further and further in trouble with each meal you eat, especially the protein meals.

You may ask: What are clean meats? Those not contaminated or treated with chemicals? You must find your own source or rely on someone who says he has a good source. Natural farmers are currently trying to organize so they can protect the name and concept of organic and natural production.

I tend to believe that diseases and conditions in the body can be handled better and faster when protein is temporarily removed from the diet, which is limited to what I call the mono or duo diet, for two weeks. This means eight meals per day of carrot juice, grapes, or grapefruit and celery. This is an overall cleansing diet of great value. I cannot claim that fibroid tumors melt away under this program. At the same time, the fibroid will not regress while consuming a high protein diet either. However, outlining a diet for a specific situation should be done only on a personal basis. In my experience, there is no diet for this or that condition; they must be individualized. This is done after an extensive metabolic survey of the patient.

Liver as Food

Q. *On 1/30/70, Life Magazine published on the editorial page, "Why John Pekkanen gave up eating liver." He claims that he has not eaten liver in years as this is where*

*animals detoxify poisons such as pesticides and that is
where the poisons accumulate.*

*I have a hard enough time getting my husband to eat
liver and if this fellow makes sense or not, I am not the
judge. Please, would you reply to this as soon as possible?*—G.M.S., Valhalla, N.Y.

A. Liver is an excellent food. It contains all the essential nutritional elements in a goodly supply. There is no
doubt that it can be of assistance in aiding one to recover
from disease and can help to maintain good health.

But! But! There *is* a catch to it. The liver is also the detoxifying organ for the cow or lamb or chicken or whatever. The older the animal, the more saturated the liver
becomes with the toxic waste products it is unable to excrete from the body. These animals cannot help but become victims of insecticides, smog, poisoned foods and
water, plus all the other pollutants in the environment today. They are no different from us except that we, as a
race, deliberately poison ourselves, whereas animals will
naturally avoid certain contaminated areas and foods if
given the natural freedom to do so. Unfortunately, they
seldom are.

As for me, I will continue to take raw liver tissue extract tablets* which have most of the contaminants removed, because they are defatted.

Desiccated liver, in tablet and powder form, from areas
in the Argentine where sprays are forbidden, is available
in health food stores. This is considered safe and pesticide-free. Desiccated means heat-dried at a very low temperature.

Carotene

Q. *Can you tell me if a person gets too much carotene
if he drinks one quart of carrot juice a day. I understand
if your skin turns yellow that it's a sign of the poisons
coming out of the body.*—Mrs. H.W., Medford, Oregon.

A. Persistent drinking of a quart of carrot juice daily
will probably cause most of us to become "jaundiced."

*See Product Information.

Naturally, orthodoxy considers this to be the result of liver damage. However, this is not so. You are correct in suspecting that this is the result of excess carotene in the skin as a result of the detoxification processes. How to prove this: Just continue the intake of carrot juice and eventually the "jaundice" will go away. Another way to prove the nonliver damage nature of this type of jaundice, is to take various tests which measure liver damage. You will find them all to be within normal range.

Raw Milk

Q. *Exactly how safe is certified raw cow's milk? Does the fact that it is "certified raw" mean that it is perfectly safe for regular (1 or 2 quarts daily) human consumption, or does one still run the risk of occasional food poisoning from drinking it?*—C.R.W., Philadelphia, Pa.

A. Certified milk is the safest milk to drink. It is not the same as milk from a backyard cow. It is rigidly and medically supervised. However, the term "safe" must be defined as to bacteria count, enzyme content and effect on health.

You will find that the bacteria count of certified milk is very, very low, while the bacteria count of milk to be pasteurized may be very high. Very "dirty" milk can be used for pasteurization, because the bacteria are killed in the process. Raw milk will sour, while pasteurized milk will rot, rather than turn sour. Sour certified raw milk is still a good food.

If you are talking about milk being safe in regard to its enzyme content, then you wish to have milk with the highest enzyme count, because lack of enzymes in the system leads to diseased states. Raw milk will be much more saturated with enzymes than the pasteurized milk. In fact, the degree of pasteurization is measured by the amount of enzymes destroyed in the process. Thus, if you are thinking of safety in terms of health and prevention of disease, there is no doubt that the raw milk is safer.

It is my opinion that if you are drinking one to two quarts of milk daily, you are asking for trouble. Milk neutralizes hydrochloric acid in the stomach and thus interferes with proper digestion, not only in the stomach, but also in the lower intestinal tract. I would strongly urge you to reevaluate your habit pattern.

Honey for Diabetics

Q. *In your opinion, can most diabetics tolerate tupelo honey when they cannot tolerate other honeys?*—M.A., Canton, Ohio.

A. Tupelo honey is that type of honey which the bees extract from the tupelo flower which grows primarily in the Everglades of Florida. It is a very valuable nutritional food because its sugar component is mostly levulose. Most other honeys are higher in glucose and not as high in levulose. As a high-levulose food, it should be relatively well tolerated by diabetics and by their counterpart, hypoglycemics or low blood sugar people.

I believe that tupelo honey and other natural sugars do not cause diabetes or low blood sugar, but that once the condition does exist, it can be perpetuated by such foods. Though this honey cannot make you develop these sugar problems, it certainly can perpetuate such disorders if you are already subject to them.

In my treatment program, I do not allow my patients to indulge in honey, even tupelo, until about six months after their condition is under control. It is then usually safe to allow them to use it to a limited degree.

Yeast

Q. *Recently my husband read about yeast and how good it is for nutrition. Now he wonders about the yeast in beer and would like to know if that is the same yeast, and which beer contains most of it. He is really interested in this question since he would not mind getting some of his nutrients by drinking beer. Could you please give us an answer?*—C.M., Orchard Lake Village, Michigan.

A. Brewer's yeast is an excellent source of nutritional elements, especially the Vitamin-B complex. It is the material used in the production of beer but is not in the beer. Sorry, you cannot use drinking beer as an excuse for a search for the B complex. It should be taken in powdered form, added to juices or water.

Table Salt

Q. *I am under the impression that sodium chloride should be balanced with potassium. Would a combination of potassium chloride and powdered kelp be advantageous as table salt?*—B.H., Iowa City, Iowa.

A. Table salt is something that should not be eaten by anyone! It is one of those things created by man. It is extracted from sea water by heat for the most part, and the rest of the minerals are thrown away. The sodium chloride is then mixed with some other chemical which will cause it to flow even when it rains. The mixture is melted at a very high temperature and allowed to recrystallize. This is what we use as table salt. Potassium chloride is a very bitter and strong-tasting substance and would not enhance the taste of food. Your best bet is to get whole sea salt. This preparation, if prepared without heat, contains many of the trace minerals. Kelp is a wonderful preparation. It, too, contains all the trace minerals with the added amount of iodine, which has been extracted and concentrated from the sea water. This substance prevents many types of thyroid disease.

Monosodium Glutamate

Q. *Is monosodium glutamate a chemical, and if it is biochemical, what is it derived from? Is it beneficial to the health of the body, as some claim, or is it harmful?*

I read that it is a brain food, that it revitalizes the brain and helps folks who are forgetful. If so, in what proportions would one use it?—Mrs. M.P., San Diego, Calif.

A. Little needs to be said about monosodium glutamate since all the recent publicity about its toxicity. I do wish to state that the fact that the name sounds similar to something that is good does not also make it good. Glutamic acid, one of the amino acids, *is* a good product and does have a beneficial effect on some brain syndromes. In Mongoloid children, some studies indicate that glutamic acid is very valuable and can make a totally dependent child or person into a relatively self-sustaining individual.

The chemists also use some "sneaky" names to cover the chemical nature of certain compounds. For example, the name of sorbic acid sounds pretty safe because it is close to ascorbic acid. In fact, some may think that there was simply a misprint on the label and that ascorbic acid was really meant. Don't allow the manufacturers to confuse you.

Freezing of Supplements

Q. *Is it all right to keep raw seeds and nuts and some food supplements in the freezer? I would like to buy lecithin granules and capsules of germ oils and Vitamins A, D and E in large quantities (10 pounds and 1000 capsules) and use a small portion at a time, freezing the rest to prevent rancidity.*—C.R.W., Philadelphia, Pa.

A. The process of freezing is a very valuable way to store various foods. There is only one big factor which must be considered and that is that the precursor to Vitamin K is destroyed by freezing. If you ate nothing but frozen foods, you would develop a Vitamin K deficiency.

One other point of great importance is that freezing does not necessarily prevent rancidity of certain oils. Wheat germ oil is a good example of this. I do not think one can consume wheat germ oil which is open to the air rapidly enough, even with adequate refrigeration, to prevent the development of rancid oils.

Enzyme Destruction

Q. *Our area Home Advisor says blanching green beans in boiling water before freezing them destroys the enzymes, thereby preventing the loss of color, flavor and nutritive value. She says that if enzymes are not destroyed, the beans will continue to mature and the quality will not be* *good. How can the destruction of enzymes protect nutritive value?*—Mrs. J.W., Chico, Calif.

A. Enzymes are very heat labile. They are almost completely destroyed by a temperature of 120 degrees, which is lower than the temperature of the water coming from your hot water tank. If enzymes are destroyed, then the food will keep. It is the enzymes which cause the food to spoil. Naturally, if the food is blanched and kept from spoiling, the remaining nutritive value will be preserved, but there will not be enzymes present. It is felt by some that it is better to have a part of the nutritive value than none.

Frankly, I do not agree with this philosophy unless it is a matter of utmost emergency. I believe in the fresh, raw foods with the least amount of processing possible. Everything is relative, and the basic facts must be faced before making across-the-board answers. If there is nothing else available at that particular time and place, then the use of these foods is allowable. But only for the emergency.

Acid-Alkaline Diet

Q. *Would you please give a simple explanation of acid-and-alkaline diet control of the body. I have never met one layman who could explain this to me clearly. Also, tell how to test the urine with nitrazine papers.*

I recently had a terrific case of canker. My tongue continues to be a little sore, more so at one time than another. I am wondering if an acid or alkaline condition could cause this.—A.K.P., Bountiful, Utah.

A. If you ever come across a good, simple explanation of the acid-alkaline balance in the body, be sure to let *me* know. Three factors come to mind when I think about these problems.

One goes like this: When one is ill, the acid-base ratio is disturbed. If it is on the alkaline side, the use of hydrochloric acid will bring it back to normal. If it is on the acid side, hydrochloric acid will bring it back to normal. This may sound paradoxical, so I shall explain. In the first instance, acid naturally neutralizes alkalinity. Acidosis is an accumulation of ABNORMAL acids in the system. These abnormal acids are certain metabolic intermediate products which accumulate in excess sufficient to cause acidosis. Hydrochloric acid helps to complete the metabolic process and thus eliminates the accumulation of the excess of abnormal acids. Both acidosis and alkalosis are helped to approach normal by the use of hydrochloric acid.

Hydrochloric acid is administered both by mouth (in the form of tablets or dilute acid) and intravenously (in the form of sterile 1:1000 solution of the acid). I usually give this solution intravenously, along with an equal or greater amount of other items so that the dilution becomes approximately 1:2000. There are no adverse reactions to this method. Hydrochloric acid is the only inorganic acid which is normally present in the system. Its presence in adequate amounts is of paramount importance to good health.

The second approach is to use vinegar. I recommend either apple cider or wine vinegar to be taken with each meal. The amount will vary with each person, but one to four tablespoonfuls in a glassful of water to be sipped with each meal is usually effective. This improves the acid status of the stomach and thus helps to digest the food. With the improvement in digestion, ultimately, there is more acid produced by the stomach. It is a treatment which eventually causes an improvement in physiology. I consider this goldplated advice for my patients.

The third approach is the use of minerals. The alkaline ash trace minerals (potassium, sodium, calcium, magnesium) are especially important. When one has an adequacy of the alkaline ash trace minerals in his system, all body functions perform a little better. Ultimately, there is an improvement in the digestion. When this happens, there is better health, and as a corollary, there is proper acid-base balance.

Nutritional Yeast

Q. *For the past three and one-half years I have been trying to introduce nutritional yeast into my daily diet without success. The same problem of extreme flatulence and gastric discomfort occurs when I take any multi-vita-*

min capsule where the B complex is derived from yeast. I have tried to alleviate this problem with the traditional means of increasing the intestinal flora with yogurt, yogurt tablets, acidophilac liquid and other similar preparations. I have also tried to boost the HCl level in my stomach with betaine hydrochloric acid tablets and glutamic acid hydrochloride tablets plus pepsin. Nothing seems to work and I am most frustrated because I know how good yeast is in a well balanced diet and I also happen to like the taste. Could there possibly be a correlation between yeast, which is a mold, and penicillin, another mold, to which I am extremely allergic?—E. F., New York, N.Y.

A. You seem to have tried everything but pancreatic enzymes. It could be that this is your answer.

In answer to your other question, no, it is not probable to cross different types of molds.

Vegetarian Diet

Q. *At this point I don't know whether to be concerned about the fact that my daughter is on a vegetarian diet or to join her. She is 17 years old and has never tolerated meat well. She suffered from chronic stomach pains and the many excellent doctors I took her to could not help. She is now on a diet consisting of milk, cheese, eggs—occasionally, whole grains, nuts, fresh fruits and vegetables and her condition has improved. She hasn't had a stomachache in months. Do you have any comments on this?—N.K., Whitestone, New York.*

A. A meatless diet or one that is almost so, is a must if one is going to become detoxified. I feel that vegetarianism as a life project is not the thing to do forever, but that it certainly does aid in the beginning. Some people turn to vegetarianism in self defense. This is so because there is something wrong with them rather than something wrong with meat.

Now, I know about the stilbesterol story and all the rest and I don't condone such practice. So, when I talk about meat being a good food, I mean meat that is natural meat and not contaminated with chemicals, et al.

The first thing I think of when a patient presents me

with this sort of history is the lack of hydrochloric acid. This naturally occurring inorganic acid in the system is in short supply in almost everyone. Percentage-wise, something like 40 percent of the people are deficient in hydrochloric acid by the age of 40. The figure becomes 80 percent by 60. But even young people can be afflicted.

When a hydrochloric-acid-deficient person goes on a no-meat diet, he conserves what HCl he has by not using it on the meat. This gives him relief because he is now able to digest his food better. Otherwise, if there is insufficient HCl to completely digest all the protein, there is an accumulation of the incompletely digested factors which then become accumulated toxins. Incompletely digested foods also cause the formation of fermentation products within the intestinal tract. The answer, in such cases following detoxification, is to add protein *plus* hydrochloric acid.

Hyperlipoproteinemia

Q. *Will you please discuss the liver ailment, hyperlipoproteinemia in your column? The patient, a man in his late 30s, was given a diet eliminating all animal fat and refined carbohydrates, also liquor, and was told he should not eat canned tuna fish. He was told this condition is incurable and he will have to take medicine the rest of his life to help the liver function.*—Mrs. R.E.M., Silver Spring, Maryland.

A. Hyperlipoproteinemia means: hyper = too much, lipoprotein = fat protein molecule combination, emia = in the blood. Lipoproteins are normal metabolic substances within the system and do become overconcentrated under certain conditions. Some of the more common reasons for overloading would include thyroid disease, kidney disease, pregnancy, taking estrogen-containing medications, obesity or recent weight gain, high fat diet, highly processed carbohydrate diet, peripheral vascular, or coronary artery disease. All or any of these could be involved in hyperlipoproteinemia.

It is my opinion that when this condition does exist, there is an underlying liver insufficiency even though not serious to the degree that a diagnosis can be made. When liver damage is apparent, I really work on this organ because it is so vital. I use large doses of raw liver extract, high B-complex doses, digestaids and pancreatic enzymes. Large doses of B-12 injections are also a must here. Then we must wait until the body reacts to this combined treatment.

One thing that I do not do is prescribe a high or 100 percent protein diet or a high fat diet. The major danger of the low carbohydrate diet is accumulation of metabolic waste products like ketone bodies in the kidneys. This can cause kidney failure. Since kidney function is vital to life, such a failure is important. One patient came to me after going on a protein diet to lose weight. He had succeeded in losing some 75 pounds but had also noted that his kidney output had decreased to about three ounces per day. He also noted that his weight would increase some five pounds per day unless he indulged in a daily sauna bath. He was able to maintain his weight by sauna bathing each day. My approach to weight loss is to get patients to eat a natural, raw-fresh diet. The fat decreases and weight comes down.

Hand in hand with liver disease as a causative factor of hyperlipoproteinemia is thyroid under-function. Hypothyroidism may even be the primary factor. Even behind this is deficiency of iodine which allows hypothyroidism to develop.

Detoxification Program

Q. *I was very interested in your detoxification program mentioned in Linda Clark's book* Secrets of Health and Beauty *but I would like to know more details. How much and how does one take the items chosen for the diet?*— H.P., Takoma Park, Maryland.

A. The detoxification diet I use for the first two weeks of a detoxification program for my patients does allow carrot juice; or grape diet; or grapefruit and celery; or pineapple and papaya; or banana and avocado for the thin patients. There is no limitation on the intake of the various items taken except that only one item or one particular combination is allowed. For instance, if the grape diet is chosen, then the patient can eat as many grapes and drink as much grape juice as desired. Drink plenty, but only eat grapes and drink grape juice. This should be done eight or more times daily. If grapefruit and celery are chosen, then the grapefruit should be peeled and eaten as an orange.

The basic secret of the diet is to start eating before you get hungry in the morning and to keep ahead of hunger all day. Otherwise, once hunger sets in, the going gets rough. Therefore, avoid hunger whenever possible. Then look at each day as one at a time. Suddenly you will find the two weeks are passed and you still like grapefruit and celery, perhaps even better than at the beginning.

Food Poisoning

Q. *I am 26 and my husband is 28 and our respective weights are ideal for our heights. Neither of us has had a history of poor health, but we have never since had the good healthy feeling we had previous to the time when we ate some all-beef weiners we had purchased at a health food store, and within eight to ten hours severe diarrhea began occurring with a very foul smelling stool. Other packages of weiners were examined by our county health department, but no food poisoning or parasites were discovered. Since this date, we have had occasional attacks of diarrhea even after we had thought we had recovered from any digestive problems. Now we are fatigued, suffer from a lack of appetite, and have occasional abdominal cramping and rumblings. Examination of our stools sometimes shows excessive mucous and slimy evacuations. Our doctor has given us some pills which seem only to be anti-laxative; therefore, only covering up the symptoms. We would like to know if there is any nutritional means by which we could overcome this situation?*—D.D., Norman, Oklahoma.

A. It certainly does sound like you suffered from an acute food poisoning situation. It is unfortunate, but I must warn all the readers again that just because foods are sold in health food stores does not mean they are foolproof. Another point must be considered: The foods could have become contaminated. At any rate, do not condemn all such foods because of one experience, but also, do not trust everything just because it is from a health food store.

Since there was a sudden onset of the diarrhea, one can eliminate such things as intestinal parasites like tapeworms and other types of worms and flukes. Your poisoning must have been bacterial or chemical. If it were bacterial, there could be recurrences such as you mention, and they will continue until the organism is eradicated from the intestinal tract. Since you have had antibiotics, we can assume this is not the answer.

That leaves two methods of approach. One is to reestablish the normal flora in the intestinal tract by taking acidophilus cultures both by mouth and by enema. This is a prolonged program, but one that will be well worth the effort in the long run. The other method is to try to build up the resistance factor within you so that you can throw off the infection by yourself. For this approach, I would use the Staphage Lysate.* My method would be to give you a series of skin test doses, 0.1cc intradermally, on a weekly basis for a period of 12-plus weeks. This means that there would be at least 12 weeks but maybe more, depending upon your response at the end of the trial period.

Finally, you could have been chemically poisoned, followed by or because of a resulting allergy. If so, avoidance of the chemicals becomes important. Unfortunately, chemicals are in many foods, so you do not know what to avoid. Control becomes very difficult. Vitamin C and pantothenic acid help guard against allergic states. Maybe this is your answer.

Raw vs. Cooked Eggs

Q. *I would like to know if raw eggs are more nutritious than boiled or poached.*—E.W., Sacramento, Ca.

A. Raw eggs are more nutritious than cooked eggs because the enzymes have not been destroyed. Cooking destroys enzymes if the temperature exceeds 120 degrees.

*See Product Information.

This is cooler than water from your hot water heater. If you are interested in the next step, be sure to dunk the egg in boiling water for 20 seconds before cracking the shell. This will destroy the avidin which destroys biotin. Thus, you can save the biotin by dunking the egg first.

High-Protein Diet

Q. *I am terribly confused about the pros and cons of high-protein dieting. I'm one of those people who's always on a diet. To go on a high-protein diet seems to be the only way to take off weight. Yet, when I do, I have constipation plus a daily battle with myself because I feel healthwise it is not good. Can you help?*—E.T., Detroit, Michigan.

A. I am opposed to a strict high-protein diet because in order to obtain the proper amount of all nutrients, you need the ability of the body to digest all the protein. Among other things is the production of hydrochloric acid, which is necessary to digest the protein. Even at age 40, many people are deficient or even completely lacking HCl. HCl is necessary for the stomach to maintain cellular metabolism. It is definitely involved in all sorts of internal metabolic activities. The end result is the acid-base balance. This must be protected religiously in order to maintain good health.

Another point involved is the fact that brain metabolism is geared to almost pure carbohydrate. The energy quotient involved in metabolism of the brain is almost precisely on the carbohydrate level and none other. It looks like the brain cannot utilize fats and protein for energy.

When I talk about carbohydrates in this manner, I am *not* talking about man-made processed carbohydrates like sugar and white flour. These are the ultimate of foodless foods and can do nothing but cause trouble to the brain when considered as food.

Please do not think I am recommending a nonprotein diet. This is as bad as the too high-protein diet. Balance is important.

Watermelon Diet

Q. *Is the watermelon diet for kidney cleansing?*—E.B., Hemet, Ca.

A. Yes, the watermelon diet is good for kidney cleansing. It is also good for general bodily cleansing because the kidney is one of the major excretory organs of the body.

Blackstrap Molasses

Q. *Could you please tell me if blackstrap molasses helps in the cure of hypoglycemia?*—J.P., Rock Springs, Wy.

A. Blackstrap molasses is a very nutritious food. In this country today we consume, on an average, over 100 pounds of white sugar per person per year. That averages out to better than two pounds per week. Since I do not indulge in it, someone is eating my share.

Molasses is another story. Consult any food analysis chart and you will see the large amount of minerals and vitamins in blackstrap molasses (white sugar has none). It is even much more valuable nutritionally than honey.

Even though I consider myself fairly knowledgeable in the management of hypoglycemia, I do not use molasses for this purpose. I consider even this wonderful food to be too sweet to be used in the early stages of therapy for hypoglycemia. Later in the maintenance period, blackstrap can be used. The point is, first show me you can get along well without it, then you can have it in limited quantities.

Diet

Q. *Can you give me any information on Prof. Arnold Ehret's book* Mucousless Diet Healing System? *My husband has been following it for about one month and looks to be at death's door.*

Is it necessary to have three or four bowel movements a day and maybe an enema to make sure you are cleaned out? He seems obsessed with this idea. He says he has a continuous post nasal drip and feels he should have more energy. He is 40 years old and up until now had looked in radiant health.—Mrs. D.J.M., Syracuse, New York.

A. I consider it dangerous to follow this sort of diet for any prolonged period of time. In general, it is not wise to create two deficiencies in order to control one. In other words, the cause of the mucus in the first place is a deficiency in the system. It can probably be controlled by adequacy of hydrochloric acid, pantothenic acid or B complex or something else. Two wrongs do not make a right.

20. General Health Problems

Poor Health

Q. *I am writing in desperation. I am 22 years old and really messed up. At age 16 I was taken to the hospital for an enlarged liver. After two weeks of tests, I was sent home because the doctors couldn't figure out what was wrong.*

Two months later, I started to receive fluid in my stomach. Again they didn't know what caused it, but thought it might be the heart so they gave me a test. They found nothing and put me on diuretic pills. When they didn't work, a stronger one was prescribed. This has been going on for six years. I have really had it. Now my body is so messed up, I cannot move my bowels without two enemas a day. My food must be watched constantly because of sodium. I constantly have gas and feel weak. I also must watch my diet because I gain weight easily.—M.R., Brooklyn, New York.

A. Your body is drastically run down. I hardly know where to start. You need everything but it must be given to you on some sort of plan. Even though you do need everything, it cannot be just dumped into your system. Your system will use it irregularly and consequently, even though you are improving, the effect will be a derangement of the balances and so you will suffer imbalances while you are recovering. This may be difficult for some to picture. The body does not rapidly get well equally in all directions simultaneously. New imbalances occur while you are getting well even though you are improving all the time.

One of the main deficiencies in your system could easily be thyroid. The thyroid has been exhausted by this whole picture. It could be starving for iodine. The dosage of iodine needed per day is about one milligram. This can be taken in any form you wish but there are easier and less expensive methods when you know them. By mixing full strength tincture of iodine (like you used to put on cuts) and distilled water—half and half—you end with a 50 percent base solution. Take one drop of this mixture once daily and you will get approximately one milligram. Take it in a little water or on food. It takes several months for this to reach its peak performance. Taking a larger dosage will not hasten the effect. You could be very pleasantly surprised as this regimen begins to work in your system.

Even if this does make you feel better, you still need a major metabolic rebuilding. Do not neglect this.

Compresses

Q. *"The papaya is employed as more than a good-tasting, nutritious fruit. A Philippine constabulary officer once was bitten by a snake. His arm rapidly grew numb. Remembering what an old Igorot hunter had taught him, he made an incision with his knife into the wound and, instead of cauterizing the wound, he broke off a green papaya leaf and applied its sap to the incision. Soon the numbness drained from his arm and he was able to rejoin his comrades."I found this article in a magazine and I was intrigued. Do you know any more about this type of natural treatment?*—E.A., Waukesha, Wisconsin.

A. I do know that there are many different natural substances which can be used as compresses with great success. In one patient, I used the fruit of the papaya for the treatment of a deep abscess of the cheek. The next morning, the dressing was covered with pus and the wound had drained completely with no evidence on the skin of anything having been abnormal just 24 hours before. Comfrey leaf poultices help many infections in the skin. Potato, grated and applied to the wound, can hasten healing, and bread poultices were used commonly by our grandmothers for similar conditions. There are many more.

Various Ailments

Q. *There are several people I know who have pinched nerves or slipped discs in the center of the spinal column and they've used collars with traction. In one case there was no help. A myelogram test was suggested. Is this necessary and is the use of Vitamin E or other nutrient helpful in this problem? Could a supplement program, relaxing muscles attached to the spine, relieve interverbral pressure and be helpful?*

I understand Tolbutamide is Orinase. Is this correct? There was a large write-up about the side effects in a well known periodical against Orinase. Can you clear up this matter?—Mrs. M.J.K.

A. Pinched nerves near the spinal column is a common occurrence these days. It is easy to see why such a problem is important since a pinched nerve is painful and causes peripheral malfunction. A myelogram is a special type X ray which is used to determine such nerve conditions. It has definite limitations as do all types of tests. The myelogram can only determine a disc problem if it has progressed to a certain critical level of deformity. Chiropractors or osteopaths may prove extremely helpful in many cases of pinched nerves.

Nutrition plays an important role in such musculo-skeletal conditions. It is particularly important to strengthen the structure and action of ligaments to hold normal connections. Assuming all other general nutrients are available and being used in optimal amounts, then the administration of an abundant amount of manganese is in order. Manganese is very valuable in the normal function of ligament tissues. If an adequacy of manganese is present, the ligaments do a better job of aligning the vertebrae in proper relationship as well as maintaining alignment. If they are aligned properly, then there is no abnormal pressure, thus there is no pain, etc.

Tolbutamide is a generic name for Orinase which is a trade name for Tolbutamide.

Poor Health

Q. *I have a very pressing problem which I hope there is an answer to. In the past two years I have been to about seven different doctors for various ailments, digestive, urinary and rectal. I have had many tests and X rays for these problems. I have also been to the Mayo Clinic, but it seems that they can't find anything wrong or help me in any way.*

My problem all evolved from a trans-urethal resection of the prostate gland. Before and after the operation I took many antiseptic pills and antibiotics, both orally and by injection. About three months after the operation, I became constipated and also developed rectal problems. My gland feels swollen and painful with drawing sensations in the rectum and the fork of the thighs. At times I also pass a whitish fluid in my urine. I also have frequent urination.

I pass enormous amounts of intestinal gas, and I have difficulty in passing my stool. My stools are mostly constipated. My abdomen below the navel is distended and I have a great deal of pressure there.

I've tried HCl, all types of digestive aids, acidophilus, whey, etc. I also take Vitamins A, B, C, D, E and bone meal, desiccated liver and Vitamin F preparations. I eat plenty of raw fruits and fruit juices; also vegetables, but I can't seem to move ahead. Maybe there is something else that I am missing. If there is I'd be willing to try it because I have no other recourse.—R.R., Milwaukee, Wisconsin.

A. Unfortunately, your story is not particularly unusual. Maybe the details are a little different but the overall picture is not rare. It does represent a state of general debility and malnutrition throughout the whole body. Of course, there are localized symptoms which are bothering you most.

What you need first of all, is a good basic nutritional program. This should include an abundance of all the basic vitamins and minerals. It is utterly absurd to try to heal degenerated states by just giving minimal dosages. Minimal dosages of nutrients barely prevent the development of deficiency symptoms. We are geared to function on optimal levels of nutritional intake. After establishing the general optimal intake, you should then concentrate on the prostate gland and determine what nutrients are particularly favorable for its function. All glands and tissues do not need all the same nutrients. For instance, optimal heart nutrition is not the same as optimal kidney nutrition.

Some of the more important nutrients for prostate are in raw prostate tissue extract.* These are glandular substances which, when taken orally, have an affinity for and go to the prostate gland to improve its function. Vitamin F is also very helpful for the prostate tissue. Since Vitamin F is closely associated with calcium metabolism, calcium becomes an important nutrient, too. These should give you some relief in the prostatic area. Pollen also seems to have beneficial effects on prostate function.

Naturopathic Practice

Q. *In what states is it legal to practice as a doctor of naturopathy? How and where does a person receive schooling? Is there a school where a person could learn?*—G.C., Kearney, Nebraska.

A. Naturopaths can practice in Oregon, Washington, Idaho, and Arizona that I know of for sure. There may be other states, too, but I'm not sure.

One school is the National College of Naturopathic Medicine in Seattle, Washington. Sierra States University also gives the Naturopathic degree.

Write Dr. John Noble, 1920 North Kilpatrick Street, Portland, Oregon 97217 for more complete information.

General Poor Health

Q. *My mother is suffering from severe pain in the lower back. She was hospitalized for three weeks and they found nothing. She also had bursitis and arthritis. She has had three injections of cortisone but still doesn't seem any bet-*

*See Product Information.

ter. Just a couple of months ago she had a sinus infection and a bladder infection. I'm sure she must be depleted of vitamins and minerals because several years ago she had several feet of small intestine removed.

What I would like to know is what vitamins and minerals would she need to be supplementing herself for this loss of intestines? Ever since she had the surgery, she has had diarrhea and recently has taken a drug to help slow the bowels down.—Mrs. J.J., Warren, Pennsylvania.

A. Your mother certainly does need a nutritional program, because she has less intestinal tract for the food to pass through and diarrhea does exist. Both these factors interfere with or prevent normal absorption of nutrients into the system. The bursitis and arthritis are signs that there is subnormal absorption from the intestinal tract because they show the need for more calcium if nothing else.

Lots of times people are shocked to hear that arthritics and those with bursitis need more calcium since there are deposits in areas where calcium is not supposed to be. To put it simply, calcium is being deposited in abnormal places because there is not enough hydrochloric acid in the system to dissolve it for proper metabolism. Enough hydrochloric acid would not only assist in the digestion of the food in the stomach but also help to maintain proper metabolism.

Postsurgical Problems

Q. *I broke open an incisional hernia since I had a gallbladder operation. This hernia broke open twice, then the third time a mesh screen was put in to help hold it up. I had two hernias inside. It is now ten months since this last surgery. About two months after the surgery, I had pains inside where the mesh was and now it is much worse. It pinches my side and it feels like a thousand needles pricking. Would the mesh screen cause pain?*—Mrs. A.V., San Francisco, California.

A. Surgical wounds do break open sometimes for no apparent reason insofar as the surgeon is concerned. I personally believe that this incidence could be cut to practically zero by the use of proper nutritional methods both before and after surgery, especially in the hospitals. To me it makes no sense not to use vitamins and other food supplements in a surgical situation where the stresses are unusual and great.

I am assuming that you are overweight. This in itself makes it more likely for the wound to break open. Naturally, when it breaks down the second and third time, the chances of getting a good repair are greatly reduced. You were confronted with a big and important problem. The surgeon had little choice but to do just what he did, implant a screen to allow the tissues to grow into the wound area for healing.

A little imagination would confirm that the tissues could and do grow into the meshes of the screen and thence are tied down. When there is movement in the area, the whole screen will move even though only part of the muscles are involved. This action could easily cause distress. What to do about it is another big question. I do not know of a single nutritional method to help you at this stage. Of course, you should lose weight. You should be the normal weight for your body build, maybe even a little less. Perhaps the surgeon could then see something that he could do in the form of plastic repair.

Gland Problems

Q. *I've gone to a university medical center and all they could do was say vitamins were bunk and for me to stay off them. They did do adrenal and pituitary gland stimulation tests and said my glands were functioning. Our family doctor is a good understanding person, but doesn't know much about nutrition except he says I need minerals and protein. He feels my gland system is not in balance someway, but can't find just where. Can you offer any suggestions or can you tell me where I might seek professional help in the field of nutrition?*—Mrs. J.M., Wichita, Kansas.

A. There are two aspects of disease which are always present and active. The one is intensity of the infection and the other is the resistance to the infection by the host (you). These should always be in balance for your health.

Nutritional tools and supplements strengthen resistance. In your case, you apparently need emergency measures, so to speak. I think that one of the best ways to attack your problem of developing resistance at this late date is to use Staphage Lysate.* These injections could do wonders to help you develop immunity. Next, I would give you some raw thymus gland substance.* The ability of the body to develop resistance starts in early life in the thymus gland. If this gland is put out of order early in life by excessive exposure to infection and/or exposure to antibiotic therapy, then the body never seems to learn how to mobilize against danger. Among other things that can be used to enhance resistance is the use of large doses of Vitamin C. Also, Vitamins D and A come into play here as well as Vitamin B complex. I consider raw thymus, liver, spleen, and pancreas to be the glandular line of defense for resistance purposes.

Multiple Problems

Q. *I have three problems: a very low white blood count; tiny red spots on my body; and very thick cuticles which grow way up on the fingernail. The one which concerns me most is the low white count. What causes this? How can it be corrected?*—H.C., Cleveland, Ohio.

A. There is not enough evidence to really discuss this because a simple statement that there is a low white blood count does not tell me what kind is involved. However, this is a condition of major importance. Naturally, all the factors needed to make healthy blood cells should be taken. In addition, raw bone and marrow is a must and the cytotrophic extract of spleen.

Sometimes, the low blood count is a preleukemic condition. In this case all the stops should be pulled and you should get busy with all the preventive measures before the diagnosis can be established. By this I mean the complete nutritional balanced intake in optimal dosages.

If the low blood count is due to low neutrophile count,

*See Product Information.

it should respond to raw spleen therapy.* If it is a low lymphocyte count, it should respond to raw thymus.

The red spots on your body are probably due to the deficiency of bioflavonoids. You may not be able to eradicate the ones already formed but you can avoid future ones from developing with this therapy. There is also some speculation that they come from a toxic liver.

As for the thick cuticles, the only condition which occurs to me as a possible cause is hypothyroidism. In this condition, skin becomes thick and dry. Maybe it could cause a thick cuticle, too. Vitamin A could help here.

Protein in the Blood

Q. *I am interested in knowing about blood protein. How does this work in relation to positive serology tests for syphilis? What is the connection with a persistent positive serology test?*—Mrs. E.D., Muncie, Ind.

A. Frankly, I do not know how to answer this question. The presence of persistent positive blood tests for V.D. after appropriate treatment is well known, but to my knowledge, the cause is not known. In the orthodox thinking, this type of case could be retreated a few times to be sure that it is a persistent reaction. Then, the approach is to periodically recheck the reading so that if there is an increase in the titer, treatment can be reinstituted at once and the risk of further damage to the host reduced. This is the watchful-waiting act.

The nutritional approach should first include a complete metabolic survey. This would include adequate and extensive laboratory studies as well as functional tests. The individual should then be placed on a comprehensive dietetic and nutritional program. Among the most important supplements, I would include Vitamins A and C, along with raw thymus and spleen tissue extracts which are designed to stimulate the defense mechanisms. The thymus helps the antibody formation system, and spleen enhances blood cell formation. These preparations are raw tissue extracts of the various glands. They are also known as protomorphogens, maybe even RNA and DNA.

*See Product Information.

I am not certain that even the most extensive program of this nature would cause a reversal of the persistent positive reaction, but I do know that the effects, if any, of this positive reaction will be reduced or almost nullified by the proper local cellular metabolism. If local cells are in good health, then they resist disease or are less susceptible to a preexistent disease threat.

Dehydration

Q. *Just what is meant by being dehydrated and the usual treatment for such a condition? In this case, the patient drinks an unusual amount of water, and urinates just as much, and quickly, too. No water seems to be retained and, consequently, no cure. Is this bodily ailment considered dangerous to health? This person remains very much underweight. Another case: Ends of toes tingle so much that it disturbs sleep, seemingly indicating an advanced case of diabetes. Urine test papers show a great deal of suagr. So far, no regular confirmation test has been made. If diabetic, what foods should be discarded until the condition improves? Can a diabetic be cured by a good diet alone?*—M.M., Winnemucca, Nevada.

A. Dehydration is a state where there is not enough fluid in the tissues. It can be the result of too little intake of water compared to output such as urine and sweat; for example, a hike in the desert without enough water. Another answer could be the ingestion of food which does not contain enough water. For example, certain dehydrated foods can be eaten. If not enough water is consumed to cover this need to hydrate the food, then dehydration of the tissues can result. It is also necessary to have the normal intake of minerals. Too many concentrated minerals without using water can cause dehydration. A shortage of protein can also be a causative factor. In an older person, the improper intake or metabolism of protein can cause such a state. Does this person drink distilled water or soft water? (Both are no-no's.) Maybe these questions should be followed up to determine the basic mineral status of the patient. All in all, I think your answer may be in the realm of low protein intake.

The nerves send tingling sensations into the brain in certain Vitamin-B-complex deficiencies. I would guess at B-3 and B-6 deficiencies here. Naturally, the individual B vitamins must be combined with the entire B complex at all times. I do not believe in individual fractionated vitamin therapy.

You bring in the situation of high sugar in the urine. Now we are dealing with diabetes mellitus unless proven otherwise. Diabetics are known to have a tendency toward nerve problems such as you describe as tingling. This is, of course, an early sign. Yet, it still goes back to the Vitamin-B-complex deficiency. Maybe this is a part of the diabetic syndrome. I suspect as much.

What foods to avoid can be summed up in one phrase: Man-made foods. This means sugar, white flour and white rice as a starter. Margarine and other synthetic fats are very suspect in this disease. Many diabetics can be helped by eating raw diets alone. It may take many months to detoxify the tissues and to rebuild them again.

Acid-Base Problems

Q. *When testing with pH paper, what would cause my mouth to measure acid (6.2 and lower) and urine to measure alkaline (7–9)? Please explain what I can do about it. Is a daily evening enema with cold water harmful and does it rob the body of any nutrition? Also, is a teaspoon of concentrated sea water taken orally harmful?*—M.A.D., St. Petersburg, Florida.

A. The real answers to acid-base problems are not easily found. There are two ways of approaching this problem. The first is to take in more acid. It must be hydrochloric acid (or acetic acid from apple cider vinegar). This aids in the more complete digestion of the proteins. The use of alkaline ash minerals does the same thing. Both methods cause the body to assume a more normal acid-base state. A urine pH of 7–9 is normal after a meal where there is much demand for hydrochloric acid to be secreted into the stomach. If this does not happen, there is an insufficiency of acid in the system. If this occurs at other times, the situation is abnormal. It means that the body is very definitely alkaline and therefore susceptible to all sorts of degenerative conditions.

Corresponding to the alkaline tide in the urine following a meal, there can be an acid tide in the saliva. If there is acid in the saliva at other times, there is an imbalance in the acid-base relationships.

A daily enema is questionable. It might be necessary and yet it can be harmful. Maintaining the mineral balance in the system is a problem and minerals are lost from the rectum per enemas. If this is your problem as described in the above question, this is your answer: It is much more normal to control the bowels by the use of raw foods, and if necessary, herbs, figs, prunes, yogurt or flax seed or flax meal. Also, bran helps.

Concentrated sea water is not harmful. In this day, when the agricultural soils are being depleted and are already depleted, the intake of supplemental minerals is a must. I frequently use true sea and earth salt as supplements. There must be a balance between the soluble and insoluble as well as the organic and inorganic minerals. The body needs both. Sodium is an essential part of the body and is lacking in salt-free foods and diets. When the adrenal cortex glands are out of balance, salt is one of the first electrolytes to become unbalanced. I have found that the analysis of hair tells me very frequently that salt is very low in the tissues. It may be normal in the blood and urine but the tissue levels are very low. Often times even only a small amount of normal concentrated sea salt tends to correct this.

Those who advise drinking only distilled water are only telling a part truth. If they are thinking in terms of eliminating the contaminants from the water, this is good. But if they are talking of not taking in the minerals (missing in distilled water) then this is not good. Chemically distilled water taken into the system must be compensated for, if mineral deficiencies are to be avoided.

Flu Epidemic

Q. *My daughter is 17 years old and contacted a virus pneumonia which kept her in the hospital and at home in*

*bed for several days. She is much better now, but after
reading Adelle Davis' books and the World Encyclopedia
we find that we are not very well off nutritionally. Do you
have any suggestions we might follow, as we are anxious
to learn anything we can from you?*—E.L., Port Alberni,
British Columbia, Canada.

A. The current flu epidemic which has been sweeping
the country these past several months has been a rough
one. In spite of all the best known remedies, many have
become very ill and have remained ill for a prolonged
time, or have had recurrences of symptoms. The following
treatments have been used to varying degrees of success.
They are not listed in order of importance.

1. Enemas—At the first sign of the flu, take an enema
and repeat a couple of times daily if necessary, not just to
cause an elimination, but to detoxify. It is wise to use
coffee enemas (brew a cupful of strong coffee, dilute to
one pint, insert rectally and hold as long as possible). This
can be repeated as often as needed to control symptoms.

2. Vitamin C is very valuable. Take large doses—even
up to 20,000 or 30,000 milligrams per day. If large dosages are taken, be sure to chew it well to avoid some of
the bloating which is almost unavoidable. Always add one
calcium tablet per 1,000 milligrams of Vitamin C. This
dosage should continue for several days after the symptoms subside.

3. An apple cider vinegar body rub can do wonders, especially if a fever is present. Rub the vinegar straight into
the skin of the back, chest, legs and arms. The vinegar can
be heated a little to avoid chilling. This body rub causes
acid and potassium to enter the system via the skin. You
are actually feeding the body through the skin, which is
very valuable.

4. Lecithin in the liquid form can abort an attack of
flu if taken early enough. I usually recommend two tablespoonsful of the liquid lecithin four times daily for six
doses (for one and one-half days). If the flu is not gone
in that time, lecithin probably will not be of further help.
If you are to take lecithin more than mentioned, be sure
to accompany it with calcium. Lecithin is high in phosphorus and it is necessary to keep the calcium-phosphorus
balance.

5. Force fluids. I usually recommend clear juices as being the best. Drink as much as possible, then drink some more. Every time you empty the bladder, drink another large glass of juice. Keep the kidneys working to maximum degree.

6. Bed rest is the only sensible way to take care of yourself. This is true and everyone knows it, but seldom follows the advice. Give your body a break and it will be better able to care for you in the long run.

7. Vitamin A is a protective vitamin for the mucous membranes. Since the respiratory and digestive organs are lined with mucous membranes, it is wise to give them all the support possible in the form of Vitamin A. Take 50,000 units twice daily for a week or two, morning only, since it is stimulating.

Hong Kong Flu

Q. *Two years ago I had the Hong Kong flu, leaving me with a constant cough, with mucus in the bronchial tubes all the time. The doctor had me on cortisone until I could not take any more. I know there must be vitamins that can clear this up and heal me, but somehow I don't seem to know the correct combination. Do you have any suggestions?*—W.S.B., Anaheim, California.

A. You have general debility following the episode of flu, Hong Kong or otherwise. You need a general body rebuilding program. More specifically, you should have the series of intradermal injections of SPL (staphylococcal phage lysate).* As a starter, I would give you 0.1cc intradermally once weekly for 12 weeks, but the length of time to be used would depend upon the clinical response. I would not hesitate to continue to give these injections weekly for many more weeks than 12. This should help your body to build up its resistance to the staphylococcal bacteria which are undoubtedly present in the lungs at this time as a result of your infection.

*See Product Information.

Prevention of Hong Kong Flu

Q. *I am afraid of the Hong Kong Flu. My doctor says that the only thing to do is to take shots to prevent it. I am afraid of the shots, too. Is there any nutritional method of preventing or treating the flu?*

A. Yes, there are other methods to treat this condition, both before you get it or even afterward. On the preventive side, the most important thing is to keep your body saturated with the Vitamin C complex (this includes the bioflavonoids as well as Vitamin K). Not all Vitamin-C products contain all these factors, so be sure to read your labels. Vitamin A is also a very good immunizer to maintain the tissue integrity of the skin and mucous membranes. Naturally, one must be in good health and have an abundance of all the basic nutrients in his system.

If you should be so unfortunate as to contract the flu in spite of these simple measures, you still can avoid some of the drastic symptoms by a very simple method. You can take some large dosages of soy bean lecithin, say 4,000 mg each 10 minutes for three doses. If this is not enough to do the job, you can repeat the three 10-minute doses again in a few hours or even the next day. Two or three such dosage periods should be enough to eliminate the flu.

There is a small percentage who will get the flu in spite of this treatment. In this case, one can continue to take the large doses of lecithin over a period of days IF you include comparable doses of calcium lactate. In addition, take some natural iodine tablets from sea sponge or kelp, one tablet each hour while ill. It is necessary to note that such a dosage will eventually cause nervousness so you must be on the alert for this complication. One basic point is that you will not get nervous until you are over the flu.

Naturally, large dosages of natural Vitamin C complex and Vitamin A should also be taken along with the above-outlined routine.

Leukemia

Q. *My 23-year-old daughter has leukemia. She was hypoglycemic since a little girl but it took three years and four doctors to find it out. She married and was doing nicely until she started to hemorrhage, and her red count went down to four. Now, her white count has gone up to 50,000 and fluctuates. The hematologist has her on a new medication for leukemia. I am making her raw carrot and beet juice daily. Also, I am giving her some high Bs and Es. Her hormones and endocrine glands are all off. She ovulates every five to six months. Since it isn't a cycle, I wonder why she bleeds. Is there anything you can suggest?*—Mrs. J.F., Beech Grove, Indiana.

A. Your daughter needs all the help she can get. It would be wise to assist nature in fighting the illness while the doctors do their best. Sometimes the doctors take over without any regard for the natural defensive mechanisms inherent in the body. This is sad because nature has provided many mechanisms to combat illnesses which should be enhanced, not hindered, by therapy.

This type of illness is the "crazy bone" in the medical world today. Orthodoxy says that there is no cure for such a condition. The nutritionists simply say that the body is not healthy and this indicates some sort of nutritional disturbance present in the body. They then set to work to strengthen the natural defensive mechanisms and to reinstitute the normal metabolic functions. Usually the general picture is improved even though the immediate problem is not solved.

Your daughter needs all the food supplementation that she can possibly take and assimilate. This is just common sense; when the stress is greatest, the supportive methods should be maximum. The diet should include only the best of organically grown foods. There should be no chemicals in the food. Any chemical is a stress when it gets into the body, thus it should be avoided, especially when other stresses are present. The food should be raw since heat destroys many of the essential nutrients. These are some of the things that can be done even when we know the battle to be a futile one. It does not pay to give up too soon. If nothing else, she may be more comfortable.

In regard to the hemorrhaging, this simply is a manifestation of the lowering of the blood clotting mechanisms. It has nothing to do with the menstrual cycle. It is characteristic of the disease.

21. Heart and Related Problems

Treatment of Heart Ailments

Q. *I recently saw a news item in our daily paper which reports that the vice-chairman of the department of surgery at a university medical school, as saying "Surgery prevents strokes among aging."*

Nowhere in the article did the doctor offer the suggestion that food had any bearing on the atherosclerotic deposits he proposes to remove by surgery prior to the softening process of the brain.

When so much is known about the benefits of Vitamins A, D, C and E on the vascular system, as proven time and again by such renowned doctors as the Shute Bros. of London, Ontario, Canada, why don't our scientists use nutritional prevention programs to protect their patients from degeneration, rather than trying to correct the deficiency by cutting and sewing, instead of preventing and reversing the condition by the natural building blocks method?— E.C., La Jolla, Calif.

A. There is no doubt that medical science in this world today has made some wonderful and dramatic progress. So many things can now be done which were not even thought of a decade or two ago. Praise the Lord for this.

However, I would certainly love to get hold of some of these heart cases headed for surgery before they are subjected to the knife. I do not propose to say that all cases can be cured, but I do know that many can be aided to a great extent by nutritional methods. The Drs. Shute in Toronto, Canada, have proven conclusively that ailing hearts do respond favorably to proper dosages of Vitamin E. It is also imperative that the proper Vitamin E preparation be used. When the proper product and the proper dosage are combined in the patient, many strange and miraculous things can happen which we were told in medical school could not possibly happen. Unfortunately, most doctors still hold to the ideas established years ago.

In my personal experience, before I became "sold" on nutrition as the best basis for the practice of medicine, I had come across the idea that Vitamin E was good for heart conditions. Like a good, alert and searching physician, I tried several patients on the best product available in the *pharmacy*. After due consideration, I concluded that Vitamin E was not helpful for ailing hearts. However, I kept trying but nearly gave up because of lack of response. Then, for some reason, I used another brand of Vitamin E. The results were immediately apparent. This led me to the health food store where I found better preparations. Now I am really "sold" on Vitamin E for hearts.

Unfortunately, I am sure that this has happened to other physicians. They have tried to follow certain nutritional ideas, but give them up in disgust because they do not have the proper products to use in their own experimentation. This is one reason why organized and orthodox medicine is blind to nutritional methods. They are taught that their synthetic preparations available in the drug stores are just as good as, or even better than, the natural varieties in the health food stores.

Ailing hearts also respond to Vitamin B. For example, during my internship, I gave emergency care to an alcoholic who was suffering from D.T.s as well as heart failure. Our routine treatment at the hospital was to load patients with a large dosage of sugar, protected by insulin, in association with Vitamin B complex. In the middle of the night, I gave this woman this routine injection, which I remember so well because I had to administer it in the jugular vein, since all other available veins were destroyed due to her addiction habit. I was thoroughly razzed about my "eager beaver" approach, but the truth was that she was no longer in heart failure the next morning. My teacher, a psychiatrist, gave the full credit to the Vitamin B complex which I had given the night before.

Many times, Vitamin C deficiency can cause heart failure. Immediate response can be attained by adequate dosage of this vitamin. Vitamin F is essential for proper contractibility of heart muscle. This is probably due to the need for Vitamin F for proper calcium metabolism.

Proper amounts and metabolism of other nutrients are essential for normal heart action; for example: sodium, potassium, trace minerals, protein, fats, etc. However, an excess of these factors can cause certain problems, too. For example, too much sodium can be very bad for ailing hearts, but so can too little. Too much fat in the blood can do some damaging things, especially in relation to hardening of the arteries, but too little does not allow the proper formation of certain hormones and thus can cause troubles.

I am saying that the best approach to good health, whether of the heart or any other part of the body, depends upon *optimal nutrition*. Minimal or recommended daily requirements are of relatively little value, since these figures simply say that so much is needed to avoid death. They do not imply that good health will be attained by using these amounts. Good health is dependent upon optimal nutrition of every part of the body, day and night. Every cell in the body must be acting in A-1 condition. The summation of all the cellular optimal action results in good health for the total organism. *Where good health exists there is no disease*.

There are so many things to do for ailing hearts along the nutritional line. I have just barely skimmed the surface here.

Heart Problem

Q. *I have had a right ventricle block and am taking 0.1 milligram of Digitoxin daily to maintain the rhythm of my heart. Also, I'm taking 15 milligrams of Valium daily. First the doctor tells me that the Valium is for high blood pressure and then he tells me it is for my nerves. What am I to believe?*

What are the side effects of the above medication taken over a period of time? Could Valium cause dryness of the mouth during sleep? Would five milligrams daily, or at bedtime, serve the same purpose and eliminate dryness of the mouth if the Valium is the cause of this?—O.T.H., Cincinnati, Ohio.

A. A bundle branch block is a disturbance in the conduction mechanism in the heart. It involves nerve tissue and not the heart tissue as such. The treatment should be in the direction of improving nerve function. Digitalis, in any form, basically does not control rhythm. It simply slows the heart rate down. If slowing of the rate incidentally causes a normalizing effect on the rhythm, you are lucky, but the primary effect of the drug is to slow the rate. Actually, it is B complex deficiency which allows cardiac irregularities to occur. Occasionally, potassium deficiency can also cause arrhythmias.

Valium is a tranquilizer. It is a chemical substance. In its tranquilizing action, it can act on many different parts of the body and in many different ways. This is why the doctor gives apparently different answers on different occasions. To him it is the same answer, but it does not sound like it to you. As a chemical drug, Valium has the potential to cause side effects, as do any of the other chemical drugs. You name it, and it can be the cause. In my opinion, this is why it is getting less wise all the time to use these various drugs. Your own reaction to the drug is individual and I must answer all your suppositions with a "yes," though this is not necessarily the type of answer which would apply to all patients.

Coronary

Q. *Cholesterol readings have been a major problem for me. My age is 30. My father died from a heart attack at 51. I worry about high cholesterol and have worked hard at lowering it. Despite all the things I have tried, nothing seems to improve this problem. Do I have a hereditary or a metabolic problem?*—W.G., Miami Beach, Fla.

A. I'm not so sure about the cholesterol figures here, though. An article I read recently came to the conclusion that the extremes of cholesterol were more harmful than the median level. 200 is about median. This represents what is going on in your system. The dietary cholesterol is only about 10–15 percent of the level found in the blood. The rest is metabolic and is there regardless of the diet. Cholesterol is necessary for production of sex hormones, adrenocortical hormones and bile salts, so do not be hasty in condemning cholesterol. Elevated triglycerides more closely represent the overeating of highly processed carbohydrates like white sugar and flour. This is important and can usually be corrected by elimination of these items from the diet along with improvement in liver function.

Heart Irregularity

Q. *Recently I had a complete physical and was told that I am as near-perfect as a 66-year-old could expect to be, even though I do have a heart irregularity. I've had it most of my life and it gradually gets worse. It wakes me up in the night and sometimes lasts 10–15 seconds. I have taken 200 units of Vitamin E for about two years and, a year ago, increased it to 400. Also, I take other complete vitamins and minerals (natural). Is there anything which will relieve it?*—Miss C.R., Mountain Home, Arkansas.

A. This type of heart block is involving the neuromuscular conduction system of the heart. This is, in reality, a type of neuritis. Anything that will help neuritis could be the answer in your case. By this I suggest a heavy intake of the B complex. A 10:1 wheat germ oil fraction by Viobin contains the neuromuscular fraction. It helps to correct arrhythmias.

Cardiac Failure

Q. *I have a friend who needs advice. He is 5'2" tall, weighs 90 lbs. and is 89 years old. He had been on natural foods for a number of years. His calves and feet are swollen and lately one leg started to drain a clear waterlike fluid. He seems to be in need of a detoxification program. Could you please give your suggestions?*—R.R., Arcadia, Florida.

A. This sounds like edema from cardiac failure. Also, with the advanced age it sounds like hypoproteinemia (lack of protein). Maybe they are of the same cause. At this age, it would take a full scale nutritional program to try to reverse the trends noted. Even though he has been on a nutritious diet for several years, we do not know what this means in detail nor do we know the amount consumed per day and many other variables.

You are right, he does need to be detoxified.

Slow Pulse

Q. *My pulse is as low as 32 at times. I have very little energy when it is that low. All that the doctor finds wrong with me is high blood pressure. I am on a good diet and take liver, Vitamin C, yeast, etc. There is no health food store near me. Do you have any suggestions that will help?*—Mrs. M.O., Verden, Okla.

A. A slow pulse (known as bradycardia) of 32 is probably a pathologic condition. Rates as low as 45 or even 40 can be secondary to a long athletic history involving great exertion in the past. Thirty-two is a bit lower and I would be very cautious as to recommendations. I would have to know much more about your heart function before making positive recommendations. However, there is a product available which has a great deal to do with the rate and rhythm status of heart function. This tablet contains raw heart tissue extract* along with factors concentrated from alfalfa, mushroom, green buckwheat leaf, green peas, fresh bone flour and liver.* The proper dosage of this tablet can control arrhythmias such as tachycardia, auricular fibrillation and premature contraction. I see no reason why bradycardia would not respond to this treatment also. Certainly, you should be observed while this therapy is in progress.

*See Product Information.

Hypothyroidism due to lack of iodine in the dietary can also cause slow pulse.

Heart and Ulcer

Q. *I have a heart condition, a leaky heart valve which usually does not give me a great deal of trouble. Two years ago I developed edema and since then I have been short of breath. My other problem is I have an ulcer at the outlet of my stomach. Do you have any advice?—* E.M.F., Nampa, Idaho.

A. First, you need raw heart tissue extract.* Take enough to do the job. If a dozen tablets per day are required, that is the dosage. You also need adequacy of the vitamin complexes of B, C, E as well as all the others. You also need such minerals as potassium, calcium, magnesium, manganese and, yes, even sodium. By this I do not mean sodium chloride which is considered very dangerous. *Whole* sea salt from the health stores is quite a different story.

Another great need is iodine, 1.0 mg daily. This can be taken in the form of kelp or, more cheaply, in the form of tincture of iodine. This is the skull and crossbones preparation sold in drug stores to put on cuts. To get 1.0 mg one needs to mix half and half the pure tincture with water (distilled). (Note: do *not* use colorless iodine.) Then take one drop of this mixture in a tablespoonful of water each day. It takes about seven weeks to see results. This information comes from a chemist by the name of Ruben Wolk. It works.

Your so-called ulcer sounds like you need more hydrochloric acid in the stomach. Most of the population who take antacids as advertised over TV need acid rather than antacids. I suggest trying two tablespoonfuls of apple cider vinegar in a glassful of water to see if the pain goes away. If it does not, one can always turn to the antacid. Insufficient acid in the stomach allows bile to regurgitate into the stomach. This causes burning and taking antacids will cause the stomach to empty so the

*See Product Information.

bile goes down and the pain is relieved. But the pain can often be relieved by acid, too, because it prevents bile regurgitation.

Heart Palpitations

Q. *I have a friend who is 26 and as long as I have known her she has loved sweets. Her usual breakfast is two doughnuts and artificially flavored chocolate milk. As a close friend, it always killed me to see her eat the candy bars and "junk" so I bought her a copy of Gaylord Hauser's Diet Does It—the book that got me started on nutrition. She has improved her diet lately because she is trying to lose weight. She now takes vitamins and is on a low carbohydrate diet. However, she is complaining of heart palpitations. She said that when she ate all the sugar and junk, her heart would beat very fast and hard about 30 to 40 times a day. Since she has been on this diet it only happens about three or four times a day. However, the other night, after a small piece of cherry pie it started the hard beating again. I think it has a lot to do with her poor eating and lack of exercise. Could it be low blood sugar or something?*—C.H., Tustin, Ca.

A. Palpitations can certainly come from the ingestion of sugar. The mechanism works like this: the intake of sugar causes the blood sugar to rise; then it falls. The more rapid and abrupt the drop, the more likely trouble will ensue. In fact, this is when the hypoglycemics (low blood sugar victims) have their troubles.

Now in your friend's case, she has been off sugar for a period of time so that now when she does eat some, the reaction seems to be much worse and profound. This is why: when one learns to smoke cigarettes, he goes through certain learning sensations like dizziness, nausea, racing heart, etc. These reaction symptoms subside after a period of time. He then becomes a veteran smoker. Then he decides to quit. Then comes the temptation: to smoke again because everyone else is doing it and it looks so good. Assuming the person has been off cigarettes for a couple of months and then smokes one, the reaction will be like when he first started only it happens all at once. Instead of being just a little dizzy, the reaction is intensified perhaps even to the point of falling down. The reaction of the racing heart will be something else again.

The reaction to sugar is very similar. While we are continuously eating sugar we do not notice the reaction because we are constantly under the effects of it. When we quit eating sugar for a period of time, then eat it again, it is like putting poison into a pure body for the first time. The purer the body, the more severe the reaction.

Heart Palpitations

Q. *My husband had a severe heart attack. He has improved and has retired from his machinist job. However, he has yearly checkups with his heart specialist, but still has these sudden attacks of heart palpitations and has to go into the hospital emergency. Is there anything you could suggest?*—W.S., San Pablo, Calif.

A. Among other things, your husband needs potassium. It is difficult to get enough potassium into the tissues except by using all methods available. He should be taking the inorganic form such as potassium chloride, or citrate, etc. He needs natural forms like broths from meat and vegetables. He also probably needs the chelated forms. He also needs raw heart tissue extracts,* Vitamins E, F, C and all the others in balance.

Another basic cause of heart irregularities is hyperthyroidism. This is the result of iodine deficiency in the diet. This deficiency of iodine can cause over- or underactivity of the thyroid, depending upon who and what you are. Hence, iodine therapy can correct heart palpitations.

Irregular Heartbeat

Q. *I am writing to you concerning an irregular heartbeat. Why isn't there ever any information regarding this*

*See Product Information.

rather common ailment? For several years now I have been suffering with irregular heartbeat which is an extremely horrible sensation. It robs you of all your strength, leaves you terribly short of breath and makes you feel as if you are about to have a heart attack. It comes and goes, suddenly, and lasts from a few hours to two or three days.—R.S., Miami Beach, Florida.

A. Nutritionally, the mineral approach is basic. Calcium, magnesium, sodium and potassium are all involved in the process. Once one is out of balance, it is difficult to correct. Even, at best, it takes a long time. Maybe your dosage of potassium, for instance, has been insufficient in duration of time as well as quantity. I have recently solved a few cases like this in a very dramatic way. It was almost miraculous how they responded, almost immediately. (Not all responded this way or even at all, but some did.) I simply gave folic acid injections. Folic acid has a lot to do with proper nerve metabolism and is difficult to get in food and almost impossible to get enough of in vitamin supplements. One case which had bothered me for many months responded with a single injection with no recurrence since then.

Incidentally, the folic acid story is important to know. Folic acid is capable of controlling pernicious anemia and the attendant nerve damage if given in large enough dosage, 5 mg in conjunction with B-12. Many people were taking folic acid in an unsupervised manner. The danger was that they could possibly take enough to control the anemia but not enough to guard the nervous system from damage. Thus, the FDA cut the allowed amount to 0.1 mg per tablet so that if patients needed folic acid they would have to go to a physician who would then prescribe enough along with B-12 to prevent nerve damage as well as control the blood picture. The 5 mg potency folic acid was put on prescription. At the present time this has reached the absurd position where it is impossible to get a 5 mg tablet even on prescription. Apparently, since few doctors prescribe it, the companies decided not to make it any more. The very best that can be done is to prescribe the 1.67 size tablet so that 5 mg can be obtained by a one-three-times-a-day dosage.

Of course the cost per tablet is unchanged, making the ideal dose expensive.

Paroxysmal Tachycardia

Q. *I suffer from attacks of paroxysmal tachycardia. I am now 47 years old and have had these attacks since my late teen years—although when I was younger, they were years apart and lasted only a very short time.*—Mrs. J.H., Berkeley Heights, New Jersey.

A. Paroxysmal tachycardia is a condition where there are transient episodes of increased heart rate. The increase may be quite rapid, even in the range of 200 or more per minute.

The usual medical approach is to use digitalis as a means of slowing the heart rate down. Unfortunately, when there is no attack, the dosage of digitalis becomes an overdose and toxic reactions develop therefrom. Thus, the medical world is forced to use quinidine. This substance seems to protect the heart from reacting in such a manner as to cause the rapid rate. Again, unfortunately, this medication does not last very long in the system so it is necessary to continue taking the drug on a four-times-a-day basis in order to guard against possible attacks. This is necessary because once the attack starts, it takes a big dosage to make it cease.

Nutritionally, there are two main areas of approach. The first is to get enough B complex into the system. The tablet I use for this is one that contains raw heart tissue extract, Vitamins C and B.* I start giving this tablet, having the patient chew and hold the material in the mouth as long as possible, on a minute-by-minute basis. Sometimes I give a dosage of anywhere from two to six tablets at once. There appears to be no toxicity and the results can be forthcoming more rapidly with the larger dosages. I keep giving this preparation until results are apparent.

Sometimes, this is not enough to prevent future attacks even when a four-times-daily dosage of one to four tablets is maintained. In this case, I feel that there is a deficiency

*See Product Information.

of Vitamin E. Here I use three different kinds of Vitamin E. They are all mixed tocopherols. I do not like to use d-alpha tocopherol because it is only one fraction of the E complex which is given in large dosages. Yes, it does some good, but it also does make more of an imbalance in the total picture which must be overcome by the body eventually. The preparations I use are mainly derived from the plum pit, the pecan nut, wheat germ oil and green pea plants respectively. I find that when large dosages of something are needed it is better to use a variety of source substances rather than more of one type. The dosage here can be in the range of 1500 mg or even as high as 3000 mg daily. It takes time to cause the bodily reserves of Vitamin E to be replaced but there should be early visible evidence that the right path is being followed.

Vitamin E vs. Blood Thinners

Q. *I have read several articles on the benefits of Vitamin E but cannot seem to find the answer to my question and would greatly appreciate your help. My mother, in her 70s, several years ago developed a blood clot which lodged in her lung; she was operated on because of this. Since that time, she has been taking blood thinners (Coumadin), and Valium and Prednisone for her arthritis. She developed tremors after her operation and the doctor had her on Artane for a period of time. She is no longer taking that drug as it does not agree with her. She still has tremors, but not so severe. She has had several dizzy spells lately and the doctor is attributing this to hardening of the arteries. Would Vitamin E taken with her other medicines create any problems? She has had a tendency toward high blood pressure in the past.*—Miss M.J.W., Portage, Pennsylvania.

A. Yes, Vitamin E could cause some troubles for your mother. It could cause an elevation in the blood pressure if not introduced into the diet slowly. It could also reduce the need for Coumadin which would result in hemorrhage.

The bleeding would not be due to the Vitamin E, but to an overdosage of Coumadin. Therefore, the blood pressure reading must be followed closely while the transition is being made over to the Vitamin E.

22. Hernia

Hernia

Q. *My question is regarding hernia. Is there anything a person can do—outside of surgery—to correct such a condition?*—A.V.O., Livingston, Montana.

A. A hernia is a condition where one structure protrudes into the space which should be occupied by another structure. The inguinal hernia, usually found in men, allows the intra-abdominal structures to protrude into the canal which allows the testes to descend into the scrotum. It results when the tissues concerned become weakened and do not hold the intra-abdominal contents back as they should. They have become weak and stretched.

To the best of my knowledge, there is no nutritional method to bring these tissues back to normal once they are stretched. The original stretching can be guarded against by a proper nutritional program before it occurs, with special emphasis on manganese.

Hernia

Q. *Six months ago I had what seemed to be a mild form of hernia (some swelling, very little pain). This the doctor verified and said, in effect, to wait until it worsened (and that it would definitely worsen); then surgery would be required. I have since tried some exercise (bicycling). Also, I've taken Vitamin E (200 units per day). The condition seems to disappear then recurs. Is there some preventive treatment—vitamins, exercise, massage, etc., whereby surgery could be avoided?*—W.B., Denver, Colorado.

A. The most obvious deficiency associated with soft tissue weakness is manganese. It is possible that a well-rounded nutritionally optimal diet in conjunction with extra manganese could strengthen this condition so that surgery may not become necessary. Naturally the degree of damage to the tissue becomes the important point.

23. Hormones

Hormones

Q. *What do hormones do and how do they benefit a person?*—G.K., Sedalia, Mo.

A. The secretions of the endocrine glands are called hormones. Hormones are secreted into the blood stream and act throughout the body in a very specific manner. There are hormones from the pituitary, thyroid, thymus, pancreas, adrenals, ovaries and testes as well as other areas. The hormones which are commonly referred to are the sex hormones: estrogens and progesterones of the female; the androgens of the male. These are primarily secreted by the ovaries and testes respectively. However, both glands do secrete both types of hormones even in both sexes. And so do the adrenal cortices. No one is a pure male or female. The percentage variations cause us to be of different types.

Hormones interact with each other. Sometimes they supplement and other times they counteract. This is a variable factor, and the variation controls our various bodily needs. In addition to action by the hormones we have sympathetic and parasympathetic nervous systems. The hormones sometimes work through these nerves.

Assuming that the nutritional intake is proper, the glands will probably secrete the normal amounts and varieties of hormones. Secretions (particularly the sex hormones) decline in quantity and quality as nutrition declines or as age creeps upon us. When the doctor gives hormones to supplement the sex hormones he is trying to delay the aging process. In this day and age of synthetics, he is able to do this quite well particularly for the female. The menstrual cycle *can* be maintained for many years after the normal menopause should have occurred, but I do not really believe that this is advisable, or according to nature's plan.

Male Climacteric

Q. *What about hormones and the female climacteric? I understand you to say that the treatment should begin 20 years prior to menopause. Being male, I am interested in what can be done hormonally for the male. I understand that it is theorized that the male experiences a climacteric stage.*—J.S.R., Tampa, Florida.

A. Yes, men do go through a climacteric reaction. It usually occurs a little later in life than that of the female. It does sometimes cause hot flashes and all the rest, but mostly it has to do with fulfilling sexual function image. The male thinks he is the world's best and tries to prove it to all concerned. He gets restless at home, too. It can be treated by the administration of sex hormones, male type. This, like any other hormone supplementation does supplement only and does not stimulate normal production. One can also take large doses of Vitamin E or the concentrated wheat germ oil. Or he can take tablets made from raw orchic tissue.* This raw tissue extract does tend to allay the symptoms of the climacteric.

*See Product Information.

24. Hypoglycemia and Related Problems

Hypoglycemia

Q. *I have been under a doctor's care for hypoglycemia. He is an endocrinologist. The cause of my troubles is the autonomic nervous system. His treatment consists of prescribing estrogen. I had not been able to work for two months and there was no improvement. I decided to change my multiple vitamin formula to a special hypoglycemia formula by a nutritionist whose diet I have been following for several months. At the same time I also started taking yeast food with calcium and magnesium added. I am now taking massive dosages of the B vitamins. In these days my energy level went up, my entire body began to relax and I could sleep better. Could you tell me if there is any way to get away from taking estrogen?—* J.H., Bellflower, Ca.

A. You have made a fantastic discovery. This is exactly why the ordinary practitioners fail in their treatment of hypoglycemia and, since they have no real treatment for it except in cases for the specialists, they deny its existence. Keep up the good work. It is the abundant intake of food supplements that is the difference between failure and success in the treatment programs of the various hypoglycemic specialists. That is, if they do avail themselves of adrenocortical hormone therapy. By this I do *not* mean cortisone or any other derivative of the adrenal cortex. It is the extract of the *whole gland* which is the valuable substance in the treatment of hypoglycemia.

A substitute for estrogen is, along with an abundantly supplied food supplement program, Vitamin E. Do some experimenting. Try taking different kinds of E even at the same time. They do work together. The 1:8 concentration of wheat germ oil does a good job too. It does contain the precursors to estrogen hormones which the body can use to make the finished product.

Hypoglycemia and Tranquilizers

Q. *For years I have suspected that I have low blood sugar, although this has never been diagnosed by a physician, since all three attempts of getting even a five-to-six hour glucose tolerance test (after thorough description of my symptoms) ended up in the doctor's suggestion that there might be something wrong with my nerves or head and gave me a prescription for tranquilizers, which I dumped into the trash can. I feel my glands (adrenal cortex and other interacting glands) probably need another "PUSH" to fully recover. What can I do to bring this about?*—C.H.A., Detroit, Michigan.

A. It is a shame that the art of differential diagnosis is almost a lost art in the medical profession. The commonest prescription issued today is for tranquilizers. This is an utter shame. It simply says that the doctor does not know enough about anatomy, physiology and metabolism to suggest something positive to alleviate the condition. This also is the major reason why doctors do not want to perform glucose tolerance tests routinely on their patients: Even if a diagnosis of hypoglycemia is made, they have no definite approach which can deliver results. There is no drug therapy for hypoglycemia. If there were, this would be the most popular diagnosis in medical history. It would (and does) make them look stupid not to be able to prescribe something. In the meantime, the patients suffer. As a result, when a glucose tolerance test is given, usually only three hours' observation is ordered. With my five basic criteria for diagnosis, a three-hour test will not expose hypoglycemia in at least half the cases.

Overweight and Hypoglycemia

Q. *I am hypoglycemic and eat the recommended six meals per day with small portions, but retain and maintain a steady weight. I have to lose 23 pounds and wonder if the protein, yeast, lecithin and soy oil cocktail in the morning maintains blood sugar level all day? What do you suggest?*—Miss J.F., New York City, New York.

A. Frankly, I do not think that stuffing oneself all at one time is the name of the game for hypoglycemics. It is true that you can control certain symptoms by this stuffing with nutritional goodies. It is my opinion and one that is followed daily in my practice, that the sound basic nutritional program is more important than the high protein approach. Let me put it this way: I believe that cleansing obtained by the mono or duo diet is a good place to start. A two-week diet of grapes and grape juice, grapefruit and celery or carrot juice is excellent to start the cleansing.

This restricted diet can be followed by two weeks of fresh, raw fruits and vegetables, nuts and seeds, plain yogurt, fertile eggs, and fresh sea food. Minor expansions of the diet follow this for the next month. This is the program I use very successfully in the treatment of hypoglycemia. Naturally, to the diet are added large amounts of food supplements so that the body can begin to rebuild itself as the cleansing continues.

As an adjunct, I also use large doses of whole adrenocortical extract—ACE for short. Much has been said to malign this injection. In my experience, I have found it to be very valuable in supporting the adrenal cortex gland while under stress. It also tends to impede the action of overproduction of insulin. This, in a nutshell, I have found is the basis of a very successful treatment method for hypoglycemia.

Treatment for Hypoglycemia

Q. *A year ago I discovered I was hypoglycemic and would like to try one of the detoxification diets you describe. Could you suggest one or anything that would help this condition?*—J.W., Yorktown Heights, New York.

A. Hypoglycemia is a complex metabolic disturbance characterized by abnormal metabolism of sugar. It is very prevalent in America today. You are most fortunate to be aware of the diagnosis of the condition. In fact, many physicians actually refuse to have patients submit to a five-hour, seven-specimen glucose tolerance test even when demanded by the patient.

In principle, the treatment of hypoglycemia is simple enough; it is the application which is difficult. First, the patient should be detoxified by using a very limited diet for a period of time. Then he should be fed all the nutritious natural foods along with much supplementation so that tissues can be rebuilt and their integrity reestablished. This is not so easy to do but can be done. In my estimation the fresh, raw fruits, vegetables, nuts and seeds are the foods with extra power in them. However, supplementation is a must when the body is vitamin deficient. The body will recover with a small amount of supplements for a short period of time but for permanent results the intake must be larger and last a much longer period of time, even for the rest of the life of the individual.

I find that the administration of adrenocortical extract is quite beneficial though not absolutely necessary in the successful treatment of hypoglycemia. If used, the *whole* adrenocortical extract is a must. It is not the same as cortisone or any other fractional extract of the cortex. The whole adrenocortical extract produces none of the side effects of cortisone such as water retention, ulcer formation, moon face, sometimes facial hair, etc. It does not contain adrenalin. I usually use 1000 mcgm of the whole adrenocortical extract in aqueous form intravenously once weekly for twelve weeks. This gives the body time to begin to heal and to establish a certain amount of stamina so that it will not revert metabolically to the hypoglycemic state. Along with the adrenocortical extract (ACE for short), I use Vitamins B-12, B-6, C, calcium glycerophosphate and dilute hydrochloric acid solution. This mixture is administrated intravenously with highly successful results. It is usually given weekly.

Natural Carbohydrate Diet

Q. *I believe I read in one of your columns that you favor a natural high carbohydrate diet for hypoglycemia. If this is so, could you please give a few menus and food that should be used?*—W.J.C.F., Gatun, Canal Zone.

A. When I mention the natural carbohydrate diet, I am referring specifically to fresh, raw fruits, vegetables, nuts and seeds. These are the power foods which help to correct hypoglycemia. I do not recommend man-made carbohydrates nor specific menus.

Glucose Tolerance Test

Q. *After a glucose tolerance test and other studies, the doctor said that, primarily from the subjective reactions to the test, he would feel my son had hypoglycemia and he recommended a hypoglycemia diet plus vitamins (a Vitamin B complex, chelamins, a mineral complex, 200 units of Vitamin E, 2000 mg of Vitamin C, 1 tbsp. safflower oil, 50,000 units of A and D and 2 tbsps. daily of pro-gest, a predigested protein). He suggested we continue with our regular pediatrician and allergist while he, in addition to the vitamins and diet, began a weekly injection of adrenal cortical extract. It is too early to comment on the treatment since we just started recently.*

Of interest, however, is the reaction of our pediatrician when we saw him. He exploded and said that he questioned what standards one used with a growing child to establish a diagnosis of hypoglycemia. He stated, categorically, that a derivative of ACTH or cortisone, which he said must be what my son was getting, could only be devastating to the adrenal functioning of a growing child. He did agree to discuss the treatment with the doctor and that is where things stand to date.

Is there an essential difference in treatment with ACE, for example, of adults and children? I know that the trend now is not only for children to see "child experts"—pediatricians—but also for adolescents to go to adolescent clinics, rather than adult clinics in hospitals. Several medical centers in New York have established such adolescent treatment centers. What would your thinking be on this question? Is their treatment so different from that of adults?—Mrs. M.K., Brooklyn, New York.

A. Adrenocortical extract is not a derivative of ACTH nor of cortisone; it is the parent substance of cortisone, or an extract of the whole adrenocortical substance and contains all the naturally present hormones from that gland. There are absolutely no complications such as you mention.

A doctor can be well-meaning or very sincere, but if he is recommending the wrong approach or throws cold water on another's work without knowing the full story, he is doing a disservice to his patients. I agree that ACTH and cortisone are dangerous drugs. Yet, these drugs are among the most popular as prescribed by orthodox physicians. Since they give quick results, the doctor is relatively oblivious to the possible bad effects. Simultaneously, he is ignorant of the whole adrenocortical extract and does not wish to know about it because the medical profession has declared it obsolete.

Concerning the use of ACE in adults and children, there is a slight difference. I think that the dosage should not be quite so large in children. If 1000 mcgm is the usual adult dosage, then the child dosage should be lower. For an infant, it should be in the range of 100 or so mcgm. Maybe the period of treatment should be shortened, too. Of course, this must be correlated with the clinical condition. Remember this, a child who needs treatment with ACE has been sick a greater portion of his life than the adult who also needs ACE therapy. This makes a difference.

GTT Interpretation

Q. *I have a crazy six-hour glucose tolerance chart starting with 80, fasting, jumping to 200 in one hour and dropping to 46 in four hours. Hope to hear any comments you may have on this.*—M.B., St. Vada, Colorado.

A. The glucose tolerance test is not simply a matter of so many numbers. Just because the numbers go to such and such a level does not necessarily determine the degree or presence of hypoglycemia. Of course, if the number is so low, one can make the diagnosis without further ado. But what about those who do not have a low level? I consider the glucose tolerance test a dynamic evaluation of how glucose is being used in the body under stress. I have accumulated five criteria which I use in interpretation. They are:

1. The glucose level must rise to the half-hour and on up to the one-hour level.
2. The percentage differential between the fasting and lowest levels must not exceed a minus 20 percent differential.
3. There must be no levels lower than the low normal level for fasting specimen.
4. The usual drop from the high to the low level is usually about 50 mg percent. A steep or precipitous drop is a negative finding.
5. The one-hour level must be at least 50 percent greater than the fasting level.

Now if you will study these and try to follow the thought pattern, you will see that it is not simply a matter of the level of the sugar though this is one factor. However, it is only one factor. In your case the high blood levels in early hours of the test indicate probable diabetes. Thus, you may be both diabetic and hypoglycemic at different times. This is called diabetogenic hypoglycemia.

Dietary Treatment of Hypoglycemia

Q. *You mentioned two different radical treatments for hypoglycemia. One was a grapefruit and celery diet and the other was an alternative to the high protein diet, which I believe was: high natural carbohydrate, high fat and moderate protein. Could you please tell the public more about your personal dietary treatment of hypoglycemia extensively enough so that one could try it correctly?*—J.H., Pleasant Hill, Calif.

A. A summary of my dietary treatment of hypoglycemia is as follows: (But, remember, it is only a part of the total program but a very important part.)

During the first two weeks, the patient is asked to go on a very limited diet of a choice of one: carrot juice, grape diet, grapefruit and celery, or watermelon. The patient is to eat at least eight times daily of only one of these choices for two weeks. During the second two weeks, the diet is expanded a bit. The patient is allowed fresh and raw fruits and vegetables, plain yogurt, fresh sea food, fertile eggs, and whole, real sea salt or crude rock salt. The transition between the first and second phases should be gradual. Again the eight meals per day should be maintained. The third two-week period allows 90 percent of what has just been listed and 10 percent of meats, grains or oils. The fourth two-week period is the same except that the percentages are 80 and 20 percent respectively. The power of the program is in the fresh and raw fruits and vegetables, nuts and seeds. Good quality protein intake in a moderate amount is correct. The high natural carbohydrates as in fruits and vegetables provide the backbone of the program.

For continued maintenance a diet in the 60–40 category is probably sufficient. Some who have severe conditions may need a different ratio. The treatment of hypoglycemia is still an individual matter and every patient must be examined and studied individually.

Treatment

Q. *After reading your list of symptoms of hypoglycemia, I finally discovered a name for a difficulty of which I thought I was the only sufferer, namely sleepiness after meals, indigestion, gas, difficulty in concentration, faintness if meals delayed, bloating, shortness of breath, extreme nervousness, exhaustion after minor exertion, etc. At this point I am rather desperate. I would very much like to try your regimen for hypoglycemia but I note that you specify certain nutritional supplements by name and advise that this brand is only obtainable through a doctor. It is hopeless to look for such a doctor in this state. Even chiropractors here have not been able to obtain a license despite numerous trys. No allopathic doctor would dare to buck the system.—Mrs. R.B.S., Denham Springs, Louisiana.*

A. I cannot treat you by mail. A patient must come to my office for an examination, etc., before I would dare to give specific advice. We in California have laws, too. Actually, this is best for you since I cannot possibly learn enough about you without a face-to-face contact. If you cannot find a suitable doctor in your area, maybe you can go to one in another state. Remember, your doctor can be a dentist, osteopath, optometrist, veterinarian, chiropractor, naturopath, as well as a medical physician.

Neurasthenia

Q. *Could you please tell me if there is any possibility of a complete cure for neurasthenia? Also, are there any particular foods or supplements that might help this condition?*—C.B.M., Los Angeles, California.

A. Neurasthenia is a term used to designate nervous prostration or exhaustion characterized by abnormal fatigue. It tends to indicate an inadequate body mechanism. It is something which cannot be measured in the laboratory so carries little respect in the orthodox medical field. Yet it certainly is a subnormal metabolic response to life. Almost any sort of clinical and symptomatic picture can be caused or aggravated by neurasthenia.

It seems to me that the first thing to check in a neurasthenic is the glucose tolerance test. I find that most neurasthenic patients are also hypoglycemic. Hypoglycemia goes along with failure of the adrenocortical glands which are your antistress glands.

What I do about hypoglycemia is a long story. First there is a period of dietary detoxification. By this I mean that the patients are put on a very limited diet for two weeks: that is watermelon or grape juice or carrot juice, etc., for a period of two weeks. Feedings are usually eight times daily, or more since I am more interested in keeping the blood sugar from its excessive rises and falls. Then, over a period of a couple of months, I gradually increase the dietary intake but always avoid man-made foods such as white sugar, flour and rice, and oleomargarines and solid cooking fats. These man-made foods are the root of many malnutritional problems. Along with the dietary controlled regimen, I first of all clean out the bowel mechanically. I use here a bulk type gelatinous cleanser and some herbal laxatives. Colonics and enemata are not shunned during this phase.

Finally is the supplemental approach which is added to the program. The step is aimed at detoxification, like Vitamin C, various liver stimulants, etc. The second step is to rebuild the tissues. This includes proteins, tissue extracts,* vitamins, minerals, et al. The aim is homeostasis or a balance between and among all nutrients within the body.

To top it off, I usually give the whole adrenocortical extract in injectable form (as well as oral), SPL as a challenge and the homeopathic oxidizer injection as an oxygen use stimulator. This group of injectables are not the backbone of the program, but the enhancers. The power of the program is in the dietary and food supplements.

Most people do not get a cure, but a very reasonable level of control so long as they practice the knowledge learned while undergoing the intensive therapeutic nutritional program as outlined above. Up to a point I can make new people out of my patients who do as directed.

Pain in Ear and Nose Stoppage

Q. *I read with interest your column on sinusitis. The person wrote of intense pain down into the ear and nose stoppage. I suffered from the same thing and found that the cause of it was fluoride added to our drinking water. When I changed to bottled water, the trouble disappeared. I do wish there were more studies on the dangers of fluoride. It also caused me to have low blood sugar. A lot of articles I have read have discussed the treatment of these ills, but don't seem to be concerned with the cause. It seems to me if the cause were discovered and eliminated there would be no need for treatment.*—Mrs. R.W.M., Trumbull, Conn.

A. I will be the first to agree that foreign substances taken into the body, no matter how, do have a detrimental effect. Sometimes the effect is way beyond anything that could have been anticipated. Actually, anything that is not a food, I put into the poison category. This includes all the

*See Product Information.

drugs, the preservatives and contaminants in the foods, fluoridated water, artificially created foods, and even synthetic vitamins and the concentrated vitamins from the natural sources. All these items are not foods and do not belong in the body; the body must detoxify them in some manner. Some are more toxic than others.

This process of detoxification involves the action of the adrenal gland as well as other glands. The more of this foreign material taken into the body, the harder the adrenal glands must work. If the adrenals are not fed or fueled properly, they suffer in proportion to the shortage of foodstuff. Eventually, or sooner, the adrenal gland begins to fail and the effect of the foreign substances takes its toll, though usually not all at once. If it were immediate, the cause-and-effect relationship would be discovered more easily. Actually, the cause-and-effect relationship is obscure to most patients and practitioners.

When the adrenal gland begins to fail, this captain of the team is in danger. The signals for the defense of the body begin to be weak, or in error. The body responds in an increasingly defective manner. Among other things which get out of balance is the sugar metabolism. There is usually a rise of blood sugar, followed by an abnormal drop. It is the dynamic form of this dip which is so very important, rather than the depth of the drop itself. This condition is called low blood sugar, or hypoglycemia.

Exhaustion is one of the most common symptoms encountered in low blood sugar. Practically anything else that can go wrong with the body can also be contributed to by the low blood sugar. This becomes a secondary effect. Further complications are the result of various factors such as age, sex, occupation, place of residence, past history, nutritional picture, etc., which vary in different people. For instance, the same factors could be present in two persons, except for an age difference. In the elder, the clinical result might be a heart attack. In the younger, it could be a headache or a dizzy spell.

However, even the low blood sugar condition is not a primary condition in itself. If the tissues were properly fed nutritionally, there would be no reaction in the first place. Thus, hypoglycemia can occur only when there is a previous disturbance in nutrition or when poor nutrition exists.

Proper nutrition means the eating of all the right things and none of the detrimental things. Thus, if we do not consume fluoride and other chemicals and *do* eat the right things we will not have poor nutrition. Then we do not develop low blood sugar, or the other primary diseases, and we can remain healthy more easily.

I agree with the statement regarding the bad effects of fluorides.

25. Immunity

Recurrent Infection

Q. *So far this year, I have been on tetracycline three times for a recurring virus infection in the throat. Every time the infection seems to clear up after the drug, but now, three months after the last acute infection, I am still constantly fatigued. The glands in the neck, throat and ear area have never quite stopped hurting and I am at the "end of my rope."*—Mrs. C.A., Detroit, Michigan.

A. Tetracycline is a bacterio*static* drug. This means that the organism in question is simply stunned by the drug. The body then must move in and eradicate the infection before it revives and comes back in full force. Penicillin and streptomycin are bacterio*cidal*. They kill the bugs! Once dead, they are no longer a threat. To my knowledge, all other "mycin" drugs are bacteriostatic.

What you need is to have your resistance rebuilt and the body fortified for normal function. My approach would be Vitamin C and all the other vitamins, thymus tissue and spleen tissue along with Staphylococcus Lysate and D&L injections.* SPL can be administered intradermally or subcutaneously. In the former, 0.1cc at a dose and in the latter 0.5cc. The latter gives stormier reactions but may be necessary for results because this çan be considered a type of fever therapy. D&L is a "homemade" solution (by your doctor) which seems to have the power to stimulate enzyme reactions within the system. It is made from 100cc pure distilled water, 1cc crude liver extract (Lilly or Lederle) and 3½cc 2% novocaine. These three items are mixed. The solution is administered at rate of 1cc per 25 pounds body weight in sites of not more than 2½cc using a 23g needle. Injections can be given by your doctor daily

---

*See Product Information.

or less frequently depending upon the degree of disease and body reaction.

Staph Infection?

Q. *I have had an infection on three of my fingers for over two years. It is a red swelling around base of the fingernail and occasionally pus erupts. My doctor called it paronychea and prescribed antibiotics which I refused. It seems to be a "staph" infection and very difficult to cure. The nails of the infected fingers are now warped and ridged. My other nails are healthy and normal. I am 23 years old, female and have been raised on a pure and healthful diet. Do you know the cause of such an infection and hopefully a remedy?*—Miss C.E., Los Angeles, Ca.

A. Paronychea on the fingers is indeed caused by a staphylococcus infection. The infection tends to get below the nail bed where the nail is forming and this makes it much more difficult to eradicate.

My favorite approach is to use the SPL or Staphage Lysate.* It is a type of bacterial vaccine made from staphylococcal cultures. It is not just an ordinary vaccine but a phage lysate. My suggested dosage would be intradermal injection once weekly for at least 12 weeks. The body reacts to the injection a little better each time till finally there is enough resistance built up by the body to throw off the infection in the finger. If this does not give the results desired, I would give the injections even more closely together, even on a daily basis if necessary. Usually two or three times weekly would be sufficient.

*See Product Information.

26. Immunization

Immunizations

Q. *I am very concerned about the controversy over children's immunizations. Friends have warned me not to give them to my baby because they will be harmful to his body. I have not been able to find out anything conclusive on this subject and would like to know if there is any evidence that these immunizations can be harmful?*—T.B., Vallejo, Ca. & R.F., Menlo Park, Ca.

A. The problem of immunizations for children is a plague for sure. It is generally accepted today that immunization against smallpox is not warranted unless one has become exposed or there is an epidemic in progress.

Tetanus is a very desirable one to have in your system when you are accidentally exposed to tetanus. If you do not have the priming dosages already in your system, then you must subject yourself to a very disturbing and painful process of getting tetanus antitoxin injections which are usually made from horse serum, but can be a lifesaving measure at times.

Diphtheria and pertussis are two diseases which are very severe in young infants. Of course, their chances of getting one of these is quite small, but it can happen. Fortunately, diphtheria is very susceptible to penicillin so can be treated effectively if and when the time occurs. Pertussis is harder to treat so probably calls for an immunization shot.

Measles vaccine is not very smart to use. True, it does prevent the disease when it is relatively light in childhood and projects it into a period of time when the complications are much more severe in the young adult stage. It can cause congenital defects if pregnant mothers catch the disease during pregnancy. It should have been had in early life and then there would be no problem in pregnancy.

Polio vaccinations are really questionable. True, there

have been fewer cases of polio since the immunizations, but we know that the disease goes in cycles. We could be in a waning phase at present. Or the immunizations could have caused this recession. If the disease has abated as a result of the immunizations, one can speculate that the disease will appear in some other manner; as some new disease, perhaps.

If the body of a child is maintained in good health, in fact, throughout his life, and therefore no pollutants are taken into his body which must be eliminated, then one can afford to use these various immunizations. But, good health in a good environment these days is almost an impossibility. My answer to the immunization problem then is that you must decide for yourself what to do. There are no clear guidelines since it is a choice between bad and less bad; dangerous and less dangerous. I cannot decide for you.

Herpes Zoster

Q. *I should like to know if there is any known antidote for one who has taken many smallpox vaccinations as a cure for herpes zoster?*—J.T., La Jolla, Calif.

A. The principle involved in smallpox vaccinations is to use an attenuated or weakened strain of the pox organisms to infect the patient. The patient then suffers from the weakened type of illness and builds immunity to the stronger and dangerous type. It does work. To use these vaccinations repeatedly for the treatment of herpes zoster is an attempt to help the body build enough antibodies to the pox virus so that the virus of the herpes will be eradicated from the system. Since herpes zoster is a virus type illness as is smallpox, one can assume that there might be some effect. However, the defense against smallpox is similar to building defense to herpes virus. If your case proves to be true, then the vaccination series could be successful.

There is another side of the story: the toxic reactions of smallpox vaccinations and how to detoxify the body once they have been used. The body is prevented from cleansing itself of the virus by having the disease, i.e., smallpox.

This means that the disease is forced inward and where it externalizes is anyone's guess.

How to eliminate the bad effects of vaccinations? My answer is that the best basis of a good detoxification program is a good, general and optimal dietary. Secondly, the use of large doses of Vitamin C will tend to neutralize all toxins including vaccination effects. Vitamins A and D are extremely valuable, too. (Do not use the synthetic forms but do take large doses of A and D.) Naturally, all the B vitamins must be included in large doses in order to help the body to cleanse itself. A strong liver support program is another must. If you cannot cleanse the bowel and liver, you might just as well not try to cleanse your body. In other words, it is a total program to cleanse or detoxify the body, especially when you are dealing with questionable effects of vaccinations.

27. Kidney Problems

Puffy Under Eyes

Q. *For the past five years I have had swelling under my right eye, especially when I smile—it looks like a puff ball. I've gone to several doctors and the diagnosis was 1) getting older (am 37 now), 2) allergies, 3) fatty tissue (which usually occurs in much older women). The left eye is starting to puff, but on a much smaller scale. The last doctor suggested plastic surgery to correct the problem as he felt there was no way to get rid of it otherwise. Eyes were checked by a specialist that did not find a cause of the problem. This puffiness is year-round and is driving me crazy as it makes my eye water from the pressure—some days it's worse than others.*—Mrs. K.S., Saddle River, New Jersey.

A. Puffiness under the eyes is usually a sign of kidney disease. Maybe the disease has not progressed to the point of being diagnosed but a good kidney support program is indicated at least to see if it works. It is certainly worth a try.

My first step in treating kidney failure is the use of raw kidney tissue extract.* Large doses of raw kidney extracts sometimes produce wonderful results. On occasion, when smaller doses do not yield results, I will prescribe as much as 10 tablets once daily. The once-daily-doses seem to cause more response than the multiple doses per day program. In addition to this program for kidney support, I also use the basic detoxification program and all the other treatments indicated following an analysis of the patient.

*See Product Information.

Best Approach

Q. *Could you tell me the best way to clear up kidney problems?*—P.A., Dayton, Ohio.

A. Kidney problems are best approached by establishing a good basic nutritional program which has an abundance of all the balanced nutrients available for the cells at all times. This is important because the body does not know that you plan to eat a certain thing at the next meal when it needs it *now*. There should be an abundance of Vitamins A and C in the diet. Large doses of these vitamins sometimes can do wonders. Raw kidney tissue extract or even defatted raw kidney substance* is very desirable, too. This should be taken by mouth in large enough doses. Some patients need only three tablets daily and others may require a dozen or more. Another secret is to take the total daily dose in one dose—even a dozen in the morning, for instance.

Proper kidney function is absolutely necessary for life. You are dealing with a vital organ and this should be foremost in your mind.

Polycystic Kidneys

Q. *My wife has polycystic kidneys. In your experience is there hope for arresting this condition?*—F.S., Liverpool, New South Wales.

A. A polycystic kidney has deteriorated because of cyst formation. The cysts form in the glandular tissue of the kidney, expand and cause the rest of the kidney tissue to deteriorate because of pressure. The only possible way to cause some correction of this condition is to provide the kidney with the maximum supply of nutrients favorable to its function. For this purpose, I use raw kidney tissue extract.* This tends to support the metabolism of kidney tissue. Naturally, all the other items like Vitamins A, D, B complex, C complex and E complex are indicated as well.

*See Product Information.

Bright's Disease

Q. *A young man, 22 years old, has Bright's disease with 6 percent kidney function. They take him to a doctor in Boston who tells them the main thing they know about Bright's disease is that they don't know anything! The next step will probably be a kidney transplant.*

I notice in your column that you use the different extracts in rebuilding tissue. Could this young man be helped?—Mrs. K.V.R., Littleton, Colorado.

A. Frankly, I do not know whether this man could be helped or not, but I do know that an honest try would be in order before facing up to a kidney transplant. A transplant is a very tricky procedure even under the best of circumstances. This is a very serious matter and must be preceded by a complete and thorough nutritional and metabolic analysis. One cannot possibly know all the intricate details involved unless such an examination is done first.

Insofar as the primary effort is concerned, the most important tissue extract to be used is that of kidney.* This contains the RNA and DNA and other types of blueprint pattern materials for kidney cellular regeneration. Some of the other factors which must be considered would be Vitamin C and Vitamin A. Both of these have a lot to do with healing regardless of the body area involved.

Maintaining proper mineral balance, especially sodium and potassium, would be essential for proper control. Fluids are essential in copious amounts. Be sure not to take in anything which might be an added burden to the kidney. The most common elements are the chemicals found in the water, air and foods. A very strict mono- or duo-detoxification diet is also in order. These are all problems which must be faced, recognized and managed before the treatment can be termed successful.

EDTA is a newer approach to kidney stones. This substance can dissolve stones quite readily. It can be administered intravenously and, in animals, by mouth. Ethylenediaminetetracetic acid is the full name. It must be handled under strict medical supervision because it can demineral-

*See Product Information.

ize the body when used excessively. It is of great value when administered properly.

Kidney Stones

Q. *My husband had a very severe heart attack. He has since then made a really marvelous recovery because of strict nutrition. The problem is that after about a year or so of taking brewer's yeast and calcium, he got kidney stones. In* Let's Eat Right to Keep Fit, *Adelle Davis says that when phosphorus is much in excess of calcium it is excreted in the urine as a calcium salt and the reasons given were: Vitamin B-6 and magnesium deficiency. My husband, however, has taken both with no results. Could you tell me why this happened?*—T.C., Biggs, Calif.

A. Kidney stones are deposits of salts of various types deposited in the urine under certain specific conditions. Some salts are soluble in acid solutions and insoluble in alkaline media. In this case, the answer to the question would be to maintain acid urine so that no more salts could be deposited and, maybe, even some of those already deposited could be dissolved. The reverse could be possible, though less likely. There are different kinds of stones. Certainly some of them have calcium as a base. Others have uric acid, cholesterol, etc. Magnesium oxide is capable of dissolving some of them and it could be the ones alluded to in the sphere of phosphate stones. Having the correct balance between calcium and phosphorus is essential for good health in many other areas of the body as well as the prevention of certain kidney stones.

Kidney Stones

Q. *Some time ago during a domestic crisis, I passed several kidney stones. I am very happily married now and my new wife is expecting her first child. Is it reasonable for me to hope that I will not have a recurrence on the assumption my stones were caused by emotional disturbances prior to my divorce? Also, what can I do to pamper* *my kidneys for the rest of my life?*—G.W.S., Downsview, Ontario, Canada.

A. There is no real way of determining whether you will be passing another stone or not. Certainly, the emotional strain of having a divorce and the preliminaries are enough to precipitate the formation of a stone. However, I would state that this is not the only cause in any case; there has to be some sort of preliminary or predisposing cause. Disturbed calcium metabolism is a common cause. This is controlled by intake of magnesium. Magnesium oxide does seem to have a good effect. Chelated magnesium orotate is an especially good source and one which is quite easy to take.

You should also consume large quantities of water each day. Most of us do not drink enough water, but think we do. Certainly, a quart or two quarts per day is not too much. The type of water is important. It should not be polluted nor should it be distilled because all the nutrients as well as the pollutants are removed. Spring water is best but this is variable, and not generally available. So, the best I have to offer is to use distilled water with solar dried sea salt added: ¼ tsp. per gallon of distilled water. Plain distilled water leaches valuable minerals out of the system.

Hydrochloric Acid Tablets

Q. *Several years ago, I had a hysterectomy. A catheter tube was accidentally twisted in the groin area so I could not urinate. For 30 hours I kept telling everyone who came in that it was not working but no one would look at anything except the bag below the bed, and since there was about a half cup of urine in it, I was told I was wrong. On the second day, I threatened to tear out the catheter and when three nurses came to restrain me, they found that I had been right all the time and laughed when the urine just spurted into the bag.*

Ever since that time, I have gone from doctor to doctor trying to get over the bladder infection that followed. When one urologist gave me sulfadine, I broke into a rash all over, but I kept taking it until I went back to him. He

*didn't seem to think much of the rash, but prescribed ben-
idryle and a synthetic penicillin which made the rash even
worse and hives developed on top of the rash. I couldn't
sleep nights because the rash itched so much. I was told to
go to an allergist. Since we have only one in our area, and
he was sick at the time, I went to a skin specialist, who
sent me to another urologist, who sent me to a general
practitioner, who sent me to another allergist. My rash still
persists. I wake three or four times a night, whenever there
is any urine in the bladder, with the rash itching.*

*I have asked three of these doctors to prescribe hydro-
chloric acid tablets for the rash because nothing seems to
agree with me. They just laugh or get mad and send me
on down the line to the next doctor.*

*Will you please tell me where I can get the tablets to
help my digestion so I can at least try them? In your article, you mentioned that a rash was cleared up after nothing else worked.*—Mrs. L.L., Springfield, Ohio.

A. Well, I have learned to pay attention to what the patient is saying. There is nothing in the analysis of a new
patient which is more valuable than the part where the patient tells his complaints and his theories regarding the
causes.

No matter what, you now have a chronic urinary infection. The first thing I would suggest is to get on the regimen that is urged by Dr. Jarvis: Apple cider vinegar and
honey. This combination gives the patient a good intake of
many trace minerals and vitamins which are needed for
good health. This is especially true for the minerals because these trace minerals control the acid-base reactions
in the system. The vinegar provides acid, namely natural
acetic acid, which helps general metabolic processes for everyone. Two teaspoonsful of apple cider vinegar in water
with each meal could in itself solve your problem.

However, you ask about hydrochloric acid. Most Ameri-
cans lack or are deficient in hydrochloric acid beginning
even before they are 40. It gets worse as the age increases.
The dosage is quite variable but usually is one or two tablets with each meal. You should have no trouble finding
the preparations which could do the job in the health food
stores. Many companies add other enzymes to the acid to

aid and assist in the overall process of digestion. Pepsin and pancreatic enzymes are the most common additions.

Bladder and Kidney Trouble

Q. *I have been troubled for many years with a bladder and kidney condition, but since I have given up eating foods that contain volatile oil, my condition has improved tremendously. The "no" foods are garlic, onions, shallots, scallions, radishes and water cress. However, I still eat cabbage, green peppers, lettuce, tomatoes, and celery. Do any of these have volatile oil? Any information you can give me of foods containing this oil will be greatly appreciated.*—Mrs. S.B., Palm Springs, Calif.

A. Personally, I find it difficult to believe that this is the answer to your problem. True enough, you have found that omitting these items from your diet causes some of your distress to subside. This, obviously, makes you think that these items cause the trouble. Maybe so, but I question it.

Could it be that there is a deficiency somewhere else which allows these items to act like poisons for you? With this thought in mind, one logically sees that a patient must be completely analyzed in order to find all defects in metabolic function. Sometimes dysfunctions can be found which have no apparent connection to the complaint, yet when they are corrected, the complaint normalizes. I am sorry to state that I do not know about the other foods which contain volatile oils. Some research in the library might give you the answer.

28. Leg Problems

Phlebitis

Q. *My husband has phlebitis and takes a blood thinner.*
You stated you should not take Vitamin E with a thinner,
why? He has been doing this.—Mrs. T., Cincinnati, Ohio.

A. Phlebitis is a condition where the inside of the veins
is inflamed, which tends to allow the blood to clot there. It
is a potentially dangerous condition because the blood clot
or a part of it could easily break off in the blood stream
and flow directly to the heart, through it and into the
lungs. This is known as a pulmonary embolus.

The usual medical treatment for such a condition is to
use blood thinners so embolus can't develop. Another
usual treatment is to have the veins ligated. This means to
tie and cut the veins and force the blood to get back to the
heart via different routes. (This isolates the problem vein
so no clots can break loose and become an embolus.)

Nutritionally, one can use a solution of ortho-phos-
phoric acid to cause this blood-thinning action. However, I
certainly do not recommend self-therapy in the usage of
this material. This is too grave a situation to do any experimenting without adequate observation. Even then, how
can a doctor, looking at you while it is happening, do
anything to stop a piece of clot breaking loose into the circulation? It is impossible at this showdown point to do
anything. Any action must be preventive or planned ahead
of time. So be careful. Use your head.

As for taking an anticoagulant (a blood thinner), it is
not a question of taking it with Vitamin E. Experts believe
alpha tocopherol should be taken *instead of* an anticoagulant. Evan Shute, M.D., has stated in an earlier book
(*Your Heart and Vitamin E*): "The popular agents used

by medical men to date have been the so-called anticoagulants, drugs which hinder further blood clotting but do little or nothing to dissolve existing clots or provide detours around plugged veins. They are dangerous, too—so dangerous that it is questionable if they have any place at all in medical treatment. There is a good deal of medical debate on this issue. . . . Alpha tocopherol is a happier answer, and a *safe* one. In large doses it not only prevents clots from spreading, but often melts them away rapidly, provides collateral circulation around the obstructed vein, and seems to prevent clots breaking loose as emboli. Its effect on fresh thrombosis is truly amazing. Even the chronic case is occasionally helped."

As reported in Dr. Wilfrid Shute's book *Vitamin E For Ailing and Healthy Hearts*, Alton Ochsner, M.D., has also reported the ability of alpha tocopherol to be the best preventive, as well as treatment, for dissolving and removing freshly formed thrombi in the large veins of the legs; he has had no trouble as a result of using alpha tocopherol in his patients of emboli breaking loose in the veins of clots which are otherwise carried through the heart and into the vessels of the lungs.

Phlebitis

Q. I am 78 years old and eat a lot of fruits, vegetables, sunflower seeds and wheat germ. About six months ago I had a general checkup and the doctor told me I was in very good condition. My heart, blood pressure and cholesterol are normal. But sometimes my hands and feet are cold. The doctor says this is poor circulation and prescribed some pills which helped while I was taking them.

About a month ago, I had a very bad pain in the back of my leg, just below the knee. The doctor says it is phlebitis. He gave me some pills and told me to lie in bed, with a hot towel wrapped around the leg and the leg placed over a pillow. Most of the pain and swelling disappeared, but some remains.

The doctor says he does not know the cause of phlebitis.

Please, can you explain what phlebitis is, and how I can improve myself to get rid of the rest of the pain and swelling?—M.K., Ramsey, New Jersey.

A. Phlebitis is a condition where there is inflammation of the veins. It usually occurs in the legs but can occur in any area if the proper circumstances exist. Trauma is an excellent precursor to this problem. So also is taking the Pill.

I certainly do agree with the advice your doctor gave you regarding the compresses. In one respect, I am more specific because I suggest the use of a solution of apple cider vinegar and salt: two teaspoonfuls of each in one glassful of water. This can be compressed around the area and the whole thing wrapped in plastic and gently, but firmly, tied in place. This compress is to be left on overnight. Many times the problem is solved in one such application. If it is not, the compresses are continued for a longer period.

One of the main complications of a serious nature following phlebitis is the formation of a clot at the local site. This clot is very difficult if not impossible to dissolve satisfactorily. This is so because as the clot is dissolved, it can become loosened from its attachments locally and be freed to flow in the blood stream back to the heart. This can become lodged in the lungs primarily, but could get stuck in some other areas like the heart or liver, too. This, in the lung, is called a pulmonary embolus. You can be checked in a matter of seconds. If a clot does not exist, the compresses can do the job. The Drs. Shute recommend Vitamin E for phlebitis.

By all means read the book *Vitamin E for Ailing and Healthy Hearts* by Wilfrid E. Shute, M.D. (Available through book or health stores.) Some wonderful results have occurred after using the correct kind and dosage of Vitamin E for phlebitis (discussed in the book as thrombophlebitis). Vitamin E has also proved to be a safeguard against clots. It should not be used with any blood thinner, however. Choose one or the other.

Leg Cramps

Q. *I have been subject to cramps in my legs for many years. I know this trouble is attributed to the lack of calcium. I have commenced using eggshells ground up very fine as a source of calcium. Would you please advise me if eggshells are a good source of calcium that the system can use?*—D.R.G., Shafter, Calif.

A. There are many causes of muscle cramps in the legs. They may be caused by a deficiency of several nutrients: protein, calcium, Vitamin D (needed to assimilate calcium), Vitamin F, found in unsaturated vegetable oils, and Vitamin B-6. Cramps in the legs may be caused by vascular conditions, and these are often relieved by Vitamin E supplementation. However, if these nutrients are being taken and the trouble still persists, it may indicate that they are not being digested or assimilated, or perhaps that they are being excreted too fast from the body, as in the case of diarrhea. The use of hydrochloric acid is considered necessary to properly digest protein and minerals. Calcium is a mineral.

I do think that raw eggshell is a good source of calcium because it is a living tissue and, as such, contains minerals which are chelated in usable form. Other sources of calcium which would be good are raw bone and marrow,* as well as various vegetable sources in the raw state. Green leaf vegetables are especially high in calcium. Raw milk is also a good, and common, source of calcium.

Calcium-phosphorus levels in the body are extremely important! You may suffer from calcium deficiency if the phosphorus levels are too high. In this case, it is necessary to take extra calcium to balance the high phosphorus intake or consume a phosphorus-free type of calcium. For this purpose, I use chelated calcium.*

*See Product Information.

Heaviness in the Legs

Q. *A good friend of mine says her legs and feet are so heavy she can hardly lift them. It seems that they drag. I suggested kelp tablets a while ago and now she is starting on sunflower seeds. I also told her it probably has to do with poor circulation in her legs and she needs to exercise them more. She has a real stress-filled job in her own private office. She has been to a medical doctor about this condition. All he does is to tell her to take aspirin and wear support hose.*—Mrs. M.B., Greeneville, Tennessee.

A. It seems that your answers have been good. The heaviness in the legs is probably due to poor circulation. This can show up in at least two directions: edema or collection of water in the lower legs toward the end of the day, and/or insufficient blood inflow into the legs. A corollary to this is that the utilization of the oxygen is quite insufficient.

But one at a time. Poor drainage from the limb can certainly cause the symptoms you suggest. Since you do not mention this sort of swelling, I assume that such is not the case. The edema in the lower legs can be due to the interference in the drainage from the legs. That is to say that there is a partial block in the venous system. This causes the blood to collect more than usual in the lower legs. There is then an accumulation of the waste products of metabolism in the blood which causes a disturbance in the acid-base relationship herein as well as disturbances in the chemical composition of the blood. The net result of these changes is that there is a reversal in the normal flow of extra-vascular fluids into the blood and the fluids tend to stay and even come out of the blood to collect in the extra-vascular spaces. Thence the edema.

If there is insufficient blood flowing to the legs, there can easily be the sensations mentioned in this patient. Here the tissues are starving for more food and oxygen simply because there is not enough being delivered to the tissues in a unit of time. The legs get very heavy because of this abnormal accumulation of metabolites and an insufficiency of blood oxygen arriving on schedule.

What to do about these situations can vary in each patient; thus she must be observed by her own physician while treatment is in progress. In the first instance, the status of the heart and vascular system must be evaluated and everything must be done to strengthen it. This means plenty of Vitamins E, C and B complex in particular. All vitamins are important but these are the most important at the present. The status of the minerals, especially the trace minerals, must be evaluated, too. Protein metabolism can be out of kilter. Kidney function must be evaluated. All these systems can contribute to the problem as can the nervous system. In other words, the patient must have a complete metabolic examination in order to ascertain the proper approach to the problem.

In the second condition, where the flow of blood is reduced to the feet, one must try to evaluate the status of the arteries. If there is a blockage due to hardened arteries, the usual orthodox medical approach to the problem is to cut out the diseased arteries and to replace them with plastic substitutes. However, nutritionally, one can attempt to reduce the arterial hardening by using large dosages of Vitamins E and B-15. Included in this vitamin approach is Vitamin B-2. All of these tend to reduce the hardened substance in the arterial walls. Do not forget the value of bioflavonoids and large dosages of lecithin, too.

Finally, the third type where there is decreased utilization of oxygen by the tissues. This is essentially a deficiency disease which involves shortages of Vitamins E, C and B–15. These vitamins not only help to deliver more blood per unit of time to the tissues involved, but also tend to improve the utilization quotient of the oxygen, so that a lesser supply of oxygen can be used more efficiently, thus giving the same net result of having more blood come into the area in a given period of time.

Swelling and Pain in Legs

Q. *What causes the legs to swell a lot and ache? I had no trouble until I had children. My thyroid is all right.*

Will mineral imbalance cause the trouble, and what will help?—F.D.T., Chico, Calif.

A. I presume that there was some sort of venous damage in the legs during your pregnancy. In my opinion, this sort of damage to the veins does not occur unless there is first some damage or insult to the liver. Therefore, basic treatment starts with the liver.

In my practice, I first try to establish a balanced nutritional program wherein all nutrients are provided in adequate, even abundant quantities. The body is then stimulated to utilize all these nutrients. The effective response ratio is rather low at first but improves as the patient improves. The result: therapy ratio improves in the patient's favor. In general, my approach is to detoxify the tissues and then try to stimulate or even rebuild them as soon as possible. This is accomplished simply by providing the tissues with all the nutritional "goodies" they can use and giving them none of the "bad" items. This creates a favorable climate for proper tissue action and growth. Thus, there is some rebuilding of tissue.

In this particular nutritional program, the protein and mineral aspects seem to be most important. The protein preparation I use is one which contains all the easily-heat-destroyed amino acids* so that when it is consumed along with a normal protein diet, there is an assurance that all the amino acids will be present in usable amounts and in large quantities. Sometimes I even ask the patient to take one capsule three times daily for the first day, two three times daily the second day, three three times daily the third day and, finally, four three times daily the fourth day. Then I have the patient take a maintenance dosage of one capsule three times daily for a period of a couple of weeks, to be followed by one daily for a prolonged period.

The mineral preparation I use is an organic item which contains all the alkaline ash minerals, especially potassium and sodium.* Sodium is supposed to be a no-no if edema is present, but I usually find that my patients do better if I provide an abundance of all the trace alkaline ash miner-

*See Product Information.

als, incuding sodium, for the tissues to use. A basic dosage would be five tablets three times daily, maybe more at first. I also advise the use of sea salt, which includes all the trace minerals.

29. Lipoma

Q. *I am told that many people have multiple lipomas—as I do. Is there any known cause or any cure?*—J.S., Woodstock, Vermont.

A. Lipomas are fatty tumors. They are made up of fat cells. They are painless and benign, but sometimes become the center of necrosis due to poor blood supply. There is no concern to having these growths except for cosmetic purposes. If the lesions interfere with function or looks, then they should be removed. Removal is fairly simple because the skin can just be opened and the tumor removed like squeezing the almond out of the blanched, shelled nut. (It is not quite this simple, but it is still a simple surgical procedure.)

The cause of such tumors is unknown in medical circles. Therefore, the treatment cannot be specific. Even weight loss cannot cause the tumors to recede because the surrounding tissues will lose fat while the tumor will not. Maybe, from the nutritional viewpoint, there is some sort of disturbance in fat metabolism. Maybe there is a disturbance in the lymphatic drainage of the areas involved. These are speculations on my part. One case I have in mind seems to be improving by an intensive nutritional detoxification program along with some herb teas which tend to stimulate the lymphatic drainage of the tissues. At best, this is a very slow process.

30. Lymph Gland Problems

Lymphoma

Q. *My husband has lymphoma. He had 28 cobalt treatments and chemotherapy called leukeran. Now the leukeran has damaged the white blood cells. All the doctor is doing is giving him iron pills. Also, I must tell you that my husband has had so many infections and has had so very much of the antibiotics, he also is getting black and blue marks on his body.*—Mrs. R.L.H., Niles, Illinois.

A. One of the major hazards resulting from the administration of chemotherapeutic agents for cancer is the effect on the white blood cells. They can be knocked out so that they are not being produced in enough numbers to protect the body. This is called leucopenia. It can be very serious. These cells represent a very important element in the resistance of the body. One may speculate that this is the reason why your husband is having so many infections.

To a certain extent it does matter which cells are being suppressed. If it is the neutrophiles, one should be given much support for the spleen. This tends to aid in the formation of neutrophiles even though they are in reality produced in the bone marrow. Raw bone tissue should also be administered because this is the area of production of the neutrophiles. If lymphocytes are low, then one needs to stimulate the thymus. In the case of your husband, I would administer both preparations* just in case since neither is toxic and one can only derive benefit. Even if only a small increase is derived from the combination therapy, it is better than none. Incidentally, iron is of no value in the formation of white blood cells. It is good for the development of red cells and to prevent anemia.

*See Product Information.

255

The black and blue marks on his body are a sign that there is weakness of capillary integrity or a tendency to not clot properly. He needs to develop the integrity of the capillary system by large doses of bioflavonoids. Minerals, including calcium, are also very important insofar as the clotting is concerned.

Naturally, a basic optimum nutritional program is essential.

Lymph Constipation

Q. *I once came across the term "Lymph Constipation" in your column. What are the symptoms and how can this condition be corrected?*—R.H., Ronan, Montana.

A. I coined the term "lymphatic constipation" to try to describe a problem. The cells of the body, wherever they are, are living in a sea of lymph. It is the intermediary substance between the circulatory system and the cells. It transports food and oxygen to the cells and transports waste products away from the cells. Some of the wastes are given to the capillary blood and others are swept away in the flow of the lymph. The lymph gradually collects into tiny vessels and into lymph nodes. From there it flows to more nodes and finally enters into the venous system via the thoracic duct. This system can become sluggish or "constipated" on occasion. So can any structure or tissue. Wherever it does exist, it predisposes to congestion and degeneration of the tissue involved. In my opinion, I am pretty sure that this is the basis for most diseases.

How to correct "lymphatic constipation" is another story. I have no real answer except that the total nutritional program is a must in order to assure that all necessary nutrients are present in abundance. Raw tissue extracts* tend to stimulate the flow of the lymph. The mono diet tends to allow the body to catch up with the job of excretion and thus helps clear the lymphatic congestion.

*See Product Information.

Adenitis or Lymph Gland Infection

Q. *My 30-year-old son has developed four or five nodes or lumps on the neck gland behind the ear. Maybe they are called lymph nodes. They are hard lumps that hurt him when he moves his head. About three years ago he had just such a lump develop on the back of his neck which the doctor operated on and removed. I believe these must be caused from an infection somewhere. What would you suggest to treat this condition?*—C.R.B., Guelph, Ontario.

A. I am assuming this is a simple case of adenitis or lymph gland infection. Of course, you do realize that the source of infection may be rather remote from the site of the current lesion. The nodes behind the ears drain the area of the scalp around the occiput and up to the top of the head. Maybe you can find some sort of lesion there to account for the recurrent appearance of the nodes. Naturally, the removal of the nodes will not correct the cause of their enlargement.

I would attack the problem with the basic good nutritious diet I always recommend along with copious amounts of Vitamin C. I would also use raw thymus tissue extract.* Then my two favorite remedies to stimulate resistance. The first of these is SPL or Staphage Lysate.* My approach here would be to use 0.1cc of this material intradermally on a biweekly pattern for at least 12 weeks. I might even give it three times weekly for a four-week program. Even that could not be enough so more doses would be needed. It takes time for the body to throw off infections like this which have been around for a long time.

The second approach would be to use the D & L injection. This is my code name for dilute liver made up as follows: 100cc of pure distilled water, 1cc of crude liver and 3½cc of 2 percent procaine. This is then administered at the rate of 1cc per 25 pounds of body weight in different intramuscular injections of not more than 2½cc each with

*See Product Information.

a 23 g needle 1½ inches long. These details must be followed specifically and religiously. These injections can be
given once or twice weekly or even daily if necessary for
really acute problems which demand drastic measures
immediately.

31. Male Problems

Prostate Problem

Q. *I have seen a urologist twice about my prostate condition and have found no relief. Do you have any nutritional suggestions that would help?*—T.D., Ft. Huachuuca, Arizona.

A. When a gland or tissue is failing, it needs to be supported in as many ways as possible to cause it to return to normal. As you suggest, the intake of a totally balanced diet with all the nutrients in abundance is very important. The one added factor needed is raw prostate tissue extract. This is the nucleic acid extract of prostate tissue.* When absorbed into the system, the RNA and DNA factors go directly to the prostate tissue and tend to normalize its metabolism. The dosage will vary according to individual and condition, but I would start giving one tablet three times daily. If this is not enough after about a week to lessen symptoms then the dosage should be doubled, perhaps taken all in one dose, six, once daily. It does not take much time to see if you are on the right track and how much to take. Incidentally, Vitamin F, as well as zinc, has been found helpful for prostates. Pollen and pumpkin seeds which are said to contain zinc may be helpful, too.

Male Breasts and Other Multiple Problems

Q. *For the last six months both of my breasts have been enlarging considerably. It does not cause any discomfort, but I know that something is not right. Also, my left leg (only the left leg) swells up. It is usually all right in the morning. It starts to puff up in the afternoon and by*

*See Product Information.

bedtime, it is puffed up considerably. I don't know if this has any connection, but I get sores in my mouth often. I also have several small blotches on my face. The sores in my mouth disappear in a day or two, and then reappear. Neither of the above two cause any great discomfort. It must be something that I eat, or something that I don't eat. The question is, what?—S.B., Riverside, California.

A. Enlargement of the breasts in an elderly male is not the usual thing. You do not mention the use of any medication for the control of a prostatic problem, so I presume that you are not taking estrogens. Estrogens in the form of synthetic stilbesterol are commonly used in the steers and capons to cause them to reach marketing age prematurely. These estrogenic substances are picked up by the human consumer and they react on him. You may have picked up a significant dose in one of these foods.

They are also used in the treatment of prostatic cancer.

This sort of condition could also result from intestinal intoxication. It would not hurt for you to undergo a good detoxification program aimed at your intestinal tract.

Incontinence

Q. *My trouble is getting up four to six times during the night. My bladder never fills up and I have a hard time controlling it. When urged, I have to run with it; otherwise I wet my pants. I had an operation for the condition but, so far, the operation hasn't done anything to relieve me. I also took some pills but they didn't help either. If you have any suggestions would you please tell me?*—F.W.

A. Urgency and incontinence after prostatic surgery is certainly a common occurrence. Control usually occurs after a time and all of a sudden as your doctor has said. Some things which could help you would be the use of Vitamin F. Also, the use of raw tissue extract of prostate* is a must for this condition. Calcium metabolism is probably at stake in your situation where the urgency comes so fast that there is spasm of the sphincter. You probably need more calcium, too.

*See Product Information.

Chronic Prostatitis

Q. *My husband, at 43, is starting to have prostate trouble, taking a long time to void. I am unable to find information on how this might be treated "naturally," and we shudder at "standard" prospects. Do you have any suggestions?*—D.P.O., Sun Valley, California.

A. Chronic prostatitis or benign prostatic hypertrophy are common complaints of the male related to his age. I personally think that the two conditions are present together in the great majority of cases. Thus, there are two major lines of attack on this problem.

The first line of attack should be against the probable infection present. The infection will be resistant to any and all types of antibiotic therapy so you might just as well forget this. My approach is to use SPL or Staphage Lysate,* intradermally once weekly. The dosage is 0.1cc each dose. The duration of treatment is at least 12 weeks but probably much longer than that. This "super" vaccine then stimulates the production of "angry" macrophages, capable of devouring other types of organisms than just the staphylococcus.

The second approach is an attempt to rejuvenate the prostatic tissue. Two supplements are of great value here. The first one is raw prostatic tissue extract* and the second is Vitamin F.* The former is a nucleic acid extract of prostatic tissue. Its power is in the fact that the DNA and RNA and other factors go to the prostatic tissue where they help the reactivation of normal action. Congestion is reduced and made normal again. Vitamin F has a great deal to do with mobilization of diffusable calcium in the system.

In addition to the prepared product I use, Vitamin F is abundantly found in sunflower seeds. Pollen also has a favorable effect on prostate action.

*See Product Information.

Hydrocoel

Q. *A friend of mine has a hydrocoel on one side. He is very frightened of surgery. Is there any natural way of overcoming this defect of the testes without undergoing surgery? I read this is a sign of a hernia. I'd appreciate very much any information you can give me on this subject.*—Miss M.O., Chicago, Illinois.

A. A hydrocoel is a condition where there is an abnormal accumulation of fluid in the scrotal sac. In one sense of the word, it is akin to an inguinal hernia. You see, in the developmental course of events, the testes descend into the scrotum from an area near the kidneys down through the abdominal wall and thence down into the sac. In some situations, this canal is not closed off completely and allows the abdominal contents to come down into the sac, too. This is called an inguinal hernia. If the opening is small enough to prevent the abdominal structures or peritoneal contents from making this abnormal descent, but large enough to allow some of the intraperitoneal fluid to settle into the scrotum, then there is a hydrocoel.

To my knowledge, there is no nutritional treatment for such a condition. The only remedy is a surgical removal of the scrotal sac so that there is an obliteration of the space. If there is no space in which the fluid can accumulate, there will be no hydrocoel. As an interim measure, the fluid can be aspirated. This is only temporary because fluid will reform in due time.

Impotency

Q. *I just turned 63, have retired and am trying to enjoy an easy life. I have little trouble in obtaining an erection (sometimes slow). However, when I climax, the semen is almost nil. Maybe a few drops at most. This has been occurring for the past two or three years. Otherwise I'm supposedly in good health, i.e., play 9 to 18 holes of golf every day, take other exercises, can still jog two miles.*—L.J., New York City.

A. Impotency is a big problem in the world today. The more chemicals we consume in the food, water and air, the more likely we are to suffer from the resulting effects. There may not be enough energy left in the body to cope with the normal functions. Thus, the more delicate ones depart first. You are in the age category where this particular function is waning. Build up your overall nutrition, including Vitamins E, B and minerals galore.

Impotency

Q. *I am an active and healthy 63-year-old and feel like I did at 42. I had a slight heart attack in 1959 and was divorced in 1968 after 21 years of marriage to the same woman. I raised two wonderful children and now I'm impotent. Did the heart attack take anything out of my system that could be replaced? I have the normal urge—am not sterile, but can't produce the necessary muscular activity for intercourse. Can you help?*—C.P., San Leandro, California.

A. Impotency is a very common complaint these days. I think it has something to do with the devitalized foods we all eat and cannot avoid. In addition to food devitalization, there is contamination with chemicals. In either case, the body is not capable of metabolizing these items so they must be treated as poisons. These poisons can do damage to the tissues, usually in the form of interfering with the enzymatic processes. (Enzymatic processes are going on throughout the body at all times. There are supposed to be some 10,000 enzyme systems in each and every cell of the body.)

Your heart attack was the result of a deterioration process in the heart tissues. The same effects were going on in the rest of the body at the same time, only the heart symptoms developed first. Impotency was the next area affected, apparently.

Treatment for this condition is a total nutritional program. I think that minerals are the key to the difficulty, and that high doses of available minerals many times will correct the difficulty.

Loss of Virility

Q. *I am 41 and seem to be losing my sexual vigor for the past six months or so. Every day I take vitamins. Do you have any suggestions?*—W.M., Downers Grove, Ill.

A. You are suffering from a major disease of the times. The loss of sexual virility is a very common complaint these days. I believe it is due to the lack of basic nutrients in the diet and the overabundance of artificial and synthetic so-called nutrients. In addition, the foods are loaded with all sorts of chemicals. There are some 10,000 allowed chemicals in the diet. There are something like two to five pounds of chemicals consumed by each person in the country every year from the normally allowed food additives. These chemicals must be detoxified somehow. One of the more susceptible areas is in sexual function. The lack of energy in this department could easily be due to the overindulgence in the chemical feast.

32. Minerals

Q. *Please tell me what is the best source of minerals so that we do not have to take too many supplements a day and still get our proper amount of minerals. Also, I read that zinc is good to use for a supplement. Where is the best place to get it in adequate amounts as a supplement?*—Mrs. C.R., Chicago, Illinois.

A. Blackstrap molasses is an excellent source of many minerals. Be sure to brush your teeth after eating it. It weakens the enamel of the teeth because of the high acid content. Beets and parsley are good sources of minerals as well. These plants seem to be able to pick up the minerals from the soil in high concentrations and this includes trace minerals.

Zinc is found in good supply in peas, beef, liver, oysters, wheat, egg yolk and oats. It is also found, in less abundant supply, in beans, beets, broccoli, cabbage, carrots, dandelion, fish, lentils, pineapple, spinach and watercress. Kelp is the best allover source.

Iodine

Q. *I have become confused on the question of iodine. We have almost eliminated salt from our diet. I do use some kelp, but am wondering how much is necessary. I have had most of my thyroid removed because of a tumor. Do I need more iodine than my children and husband? Can a person such as myself with almost no thyroid look forward to a normal life span?*—Mrs. S.B.H., Burns, Oreg.

A. Iodine is needed in about one mg amount per day by the average normal person. This is about equivalent to 10 kelp tablets. It can hardly be met by iodized salt, but do not stop using iodized salt for this reason. This much iodine as found in iodized salt can be the difference between normal intake of iodine or not. Shunning salt is not good! Sodium is very important for proper metabolism. For instance, if there is an insufficiency of sodium in the body, then it becomes very difficult for the body to utilize calcium. You had a thyroidectomy. This makes it all the more important for you to have a normal intake of iodine.

Dolomite

Q. *A 28-year-old customer of my health food store tells me she has menstruated for the first time in her life last month. She attributes this to the fact she is now taking dolomite. Her doctor disputes any connection between dolomite and her improved condition. So, could she be on the wrong track?*—E.C., Key West, Florida.

A. It is possible that calcium or magnesium did complement her needs so this improvement did result. Remember that magnesium is involved in 70 percent of the enzyme reactions in the body so that an adequacy is needed for health.

I am against dolomite for two reasons: first, some dolomite has been tested and found to contain 28 p.p.m. (parts per million) lead. Lead is one of the major pollutants in the world today and I do not think that it would be wise to aggravate the problem. Second, dolomite mined in this country comes from the southeast and contains large doses of fluoride. This is not precisely the same as the fluoride in public water supplies, which is a deadly poison, but the danger remains.

Dolomite

Q. *In your recent column you have advised against using dolomite. This is very confusing to me since I have always believed it to be beneficial. Can you explain more fully?*—B.P., Philadephia, Pennsylvania.

A. There have been several questions and statements

concerning my dolomite statement and its use in humans. Dolomite is a ground-rock deposit composed of calcium-magnesium carbonate.

Dolomite is the material found in beds of compact limestone as the Cliffs of Dover. It is natural in the sense that it comes from nature, but is not organic in the sense that it does not come from living tissues. Somehow, it is absorbed into the system but in an apparently unusable form. I have seen blood and hair levels which are normal or high in persons who are taking dolomite, but who also have symptoms which are indicative of calcium deficiency. In fact, the greater the intake of dolomite the greater the apparent calcium deficiency! For instance, when dolomite first became popular, I began to use more and more calcium lactate which contained magnesium as well. The net result was that the more I used it, the more need resulted. I was able to correlate this impression with new patients who were taking dolomite. My conclusion was that there was some sort of block to the utilization of calcium even though it became measurably increased in the system. When I went back to my organic type calcium-magnesium preparation,* the great and desperate need for calcium in my practice suddenly diminished. I do not know why this is so.

As stated before, some forms of dolomite contain lead.

Abundance of Iron

Q. *Three or more years ago I began feeling tired and run down most of the time. Then, 18 months ago, one doctor told me I was anemic and with no further tests to find why I was in this condition he started giving me, among other things, 300 mg of iron per day in capsule form, a steroid compound, plus three shots per week. I was having terrific headaches and was given four Darvon per day for this. Within six weeks my bone marrow had quit making new cells and I was in the hospital for the tests I should have had before all this medication. Needless to say, I had to have two units of blood each two weeks and the tests revealed only that I had too much iron. The*

*See Product Information.

doctors say that they do not know what caused my condition and they can do nothing for me except give me transfusions which would only build up more iron and could eventually be fatal. Finding this hard to accept, I started reading and working on a health program designed to give my body the best nutrition I could to aid it in healing itself. The doctor told me this would make no difference, that my problem was not nutrition. In spite of this discouragement, I went ahead with vitamin supplements and detoxification at different times. At this time I have not had a blood transfusion since but my blood count is still very low: (Hct—28, WBC—around 3,000 and platelet count ranges from 2,000 to 18,000). I realize this is a rather long letter but thought the background necessary for an intelligent answer to my question. I shall have quite an iron buildup in my body which the doctor says is increasing because of my low blood count. Do you know of anything I can do to rid my body of iron?—R.R., Concrete, Wash.

A. Again, as in all conditions, there must be a basic approach which includes all the necessary nutrients in abundance. On top of this you need all the items which are especially needed for good bone marrow health. First, there is on the market a raw enzymatic extraction of bone which stimulates bone marrow activity.* Next, you need some raw spleen tissue for stimulation of blood activity.* The spleen also has to do with removal of solid wastes from the blood and other important functions. Raw thymus gland extract is needed, along with Vitamin T (found in sesame seeds) for platelets.

Certainly, the use of adrenocortical stimulants is appropriate because this is a time of maximum stress by the body. I do not approve of the use of corticosteroids but the whole adrenocortical extract. This has all the benefits of the corticosteriods but without the complications.

This condition requires the utmost of skill in management, but do not give up. Some surprising results may be forthcoming if an adequate effort is made. Naturally a total program is a must with you.

*See Product Information.

Calcium

Q. *Presently I have a problem of poor calcium absorption. I had been taking bone calcium for about two years, four to six tablets daily, but recently I have been getting a stinging pain in my left and right back in the kidney areas. It will smart, itch and finally get sore, and as I stop taking the bone meal it will disappear in three to four days. I have had a urologist check me thoroughly and he found nothing.*—W.E.F., La Mesa, Ca.

A. Most bone meal tablets available in stores today are cooked in one way or another. I use and always recommend raw bone meal.* This can make all the difference in the world.

Calcium Phosphorus

Q. *You advise not to take inorganic calcium and phosphorus together. I take dolomite as directed—one teaspoon daily—and at the same time lecithin daily, which contains phosphorus. My leg cramps have stopped but every once in a while I get a funny feeling during the night. The only remedy I find that helps is to get out of bed, stand on the bare cool wooden floor and the feeling passes. Do you have any suggestions?*—M.G., Westwood, N.J.

A. Regarding the taking of calcium and phosphorus at the same time, almost all natural sources of these substances occur together. Bone meal is a case in point. Vegetarian sources of calcium also contain phosphorus. Since these products do help the body in need of calcium, I am in favor of using them. I do think that the controlling force is the pH, or the acid-base reaction. Calcium cannot be absorbed into the system unless there is sufficient acid. Try this to see if the situation does not change. As stated before, I am antidolomite. In my estimation, it clinically creates a greater need for calcium.

*See Product Information.

Calcium-Phosphorus Ratio

Q. *You referred to a ratio of two and one-half parts calcium to one part phosphorus as being desirable. I had thought that the ratio should be reversed. Is this true?*— H.K., Sioux Falls, So. Dakota.

A. The calcium-phosphorus ratio of two and one-half calcium to one of phosphorus refers to the levels in the blood. This is not necessarily the ratio to be found in the foods eaten. Just because you eat something in a certain ratio does not mean that this will be the outcome in the blood. The body is an organism which does not always follow the laws of chemistry and physics. It is possible for the body, under certain conditions, to transmute sodium into potassium. Read *Biological Transmutations* by Louis Kervran (Swan House Publishing Co., P.O. Box 638, Binghamton, N.Y.). You will learn that the living body can do certain things under certain circumstances which could easily be the difference between life and death.

33. Miscellaneous Problems

Adrenal Glands

Q. *My problem pertains to the adrenal glands. My glands aren't working right or, rather, they have failed in their duty. I have been complaining about tiredness for a number of years. Lack of pep, energy. I still have a good appetite. I thought it was anemia, so I took iron tablets and ate a lot of foods rich in iron, to no avail. About five months ago I started to lose weight. I am 5' 10½" tall, never weighed more than 135, then I dropped steadily down to 110. The tiredness increased, especially if I went upstairs. My legs were very weak.*

I finally decided to see a doctor. He put me in the hospital and there I was examined, X-rayed and had blood and urine tests. They found out it was the adrenal glands causing the trouble.

I started taking cortisone pills, salt tablets (put plenty of salt on foods) and another pill that I don't know the name of, and one to increase my heart beat as my blood pressure was low. The doctor wanted to raise it and put some weight on me.

I did gain a few pounds while in the hospital but since going back to work I lost more. Now I'm down to 100 lbs. I am much weaker so the pills aren't doing any good. That is why I hope you can help me. Perhaps I have low blood sugar? It can't be I wasn't eating right because I try to eat the best food (natural) I can get; plus taking vitamins and minerals.

If I don't soon regain my health, I won't be able to hold my job. I want to regain my health and the doctor said it is going to take a long time, but I don't want to keep on taking pills the rest of my life.

I will appreciate and follow any advice you can give me.—E.S., Cressona, Pa.

271

A. It certainly does sound as if you suffer from low blood sugar. You do make one common error in saying that surely it cannot be because you have been eating correctly for some time and taking all the natural vitamins you can get. Let me advise you right now that it does make a great deal of difference what kinds of vitamins you are taking because there are great differences even when all the labels appear to be the same. Also, you probably have not used health foods all your life. Your total history is important in determining the kind of person you are now.

Adrenocortical failure is, in my estimation, as based upon Dr. Tintera's work, one of the major causes of hypoglycemia. This is due to the relative excess of insulin resulting in the system when there is failure to produce the proper amount or balance in the anti-insulin factors as secreted by the adrenal cortex. The treatment for this condition is basically nutritional but certainly is also primarily aimed at the adrenocortical glands. These glands secrete some 34 different hormones among which is cortisone. In order to adequately support the adrenocortical glands, it is necessary to supply all the hormones in proper balance. This is done by giving the whole adrenocortical extract injections. This extract contains all the hormones secreted by the cortex in normally balanced levels. This is NOT the same thing as giving the corticotrophic hormones or the corticosteroids. (There is all the difference in the world.) On one hand, all the hormones are present in normally balanced levels and on the other, there is only one hormone present without the necessary supporting members. When the single hormone is administered, the results are one-sided. You get an abundance of one type and a shortage, in an aggravated degree, of the abundant hormones. Naturally, this leads to all sorts of complications. You can find a more complete discussion of this theory in my book *A New Breed of Doctor,* now in paperback. Ask your book store.

Adrenocortical Gland Failure

Q. *A few years ago I noticed dark skin pigmentation on the sides of my face. A year ago I began taking Vitamin*

A (25,000 I.U. daily), B complex, along with pantothenic acid and niacinamide. I read in a health book that dark skin pigmentation on the face is a B-vitamin deficiency. What can you suggest?—D.J.B., San Jose, Ca.

A. Your pigmentation sounds to me like adrenocortical gland failure. This is one of the aspects of hypoglycemia where the drop in blood sugar is secondary to the inefficiency of the adrenal cortex to secrete anti-insulin factors. Even with excellent control of the hypoglycemia, it will take a long time for the pigmentation to subside.

Ganglion

Q. *My six-year-old daughter has a ganglion on her right gland, near the main artery. I noticed it about six months ago. It doesn't hurt her. Do you think this should be surgically removed, or is there another treatment? My four-year-old son was born with one testicle down; the other is high up on the right side. Would it harm him healthwise if it doesn't come down at all? Is there any herbal treatment for it?*—E.W., Kitimat, British Columbia, Canada.

A. I know of no nutritional method of correcting a ganglion. While talking to a friend last week, he mentioned that he had cured a ganglion by using homeopathic measures. We did not discuss the specific remedy used because each person differs. Maybe a homeopathic physician can be of assistance.

An undescended testicle indicates that there is an hormonal disturbance; i.e., a deficiency in the chorionic gonadotrophin. This is a pituitary hormone and is very important in this particular function. In the long run, it also indicates that there is a pituitary deficiency in the boy and that he will probably develop other defects due to the deficiency. It is important to remedy this situation as soon as possible since the action of the pituitary goes on all the time and the longer it goes on without doing its proper work, the harder it is to overcome. Your son is now at about the correct age, depending upon bodily build, to go ahead and try to do something about this condition.

Therapy should first be a strong nutritional program to

be sure that all the basics are present. It can be rather miraculous to discover that there is a deficiency present which causes such a response in the boy. On the other hand, if no results are forthcoming from the nutritional program, the use of human chorionic gonadotrophin can be tried. The dosage here will vary, but he should have a good try at this in order to have the testis descend spontaneously. Incidentally, the testis does not secrete the proper hormones unless the temperature is just below the normal bodily temperature. This is the reason that the testes are carried in a sac rather than being inside the body. A testis transplanted to the peritoneal cavity, for instance, will not secrete normally.

Finally, if there seems to be no hope from the above methods, it is wise to use a surgical procedure to cause the testis to descend.

Dr. Volf, now deceased, from Demark, used sound vibrations to cure such problems. He used high intensity sound to cause certain central nervous system reactions to become more normal and sometimes the testes would descend normally.

Huntington's Disease

Q. *I have several relatives and friends with Huntington's disease. Orthodox medicine offers no hope for this unusual condition. Do you know of any possible nutritional means of help for it?*—J.W., San Diego, Ca.

A. After damage is done to tissues, especially neurological tissue, the chances of correcting the condition are greatly reduced. In any event, the nutritional practice should not be directed toward the disease but to the person. Many people have the same underlying causative factors but the external manifestations vary according to their sex, age, nationality, early habit patterns, etc. Thus, people must be treated as individuals rather than as conditions.

Factor V Deficiency

Q. *I have a friend who is a para-hemophiliac. She has so-called factor V deficiency. What would be the indicated nutritional remedy?*—R.O., Alameda, Ca.

A. Factor V is an hereditary factor necessary for the coagulation of blood. Hemophilia can be the result of several different factors being missing like VIII, IX, XI, etc., all hereditary factors. This means that there is nothing which can be done for them. It is like being born without an arm.

Amnesia

Q. *Two years ago I had my first experience with amnesia. The doctor advised my husband not to be too concerned as it would last but a few hours. This spring—just two years later, I had my second experience with it. I left in our car to keep an appointment, and was home one hour later not knowing where I had been and not keeping my appointment. I am quite concerned because I do drive the children to different places and although I drove safely home the last time, could it become dangerous?*—Mrs. E.M., Galveston, Indiana.

A. Amnesia is generally precipitated by an emotional crisis, but not always. In any event, it is always the result of the combination of the stress plus a crisis of some sort.

One of the most important stress factors in this type of illness is the nutritional status of the nervous system. The primary nutrients which can help are B-3 (niacin), B-6 and C, commonly accepted factors of megavitamin therapy. Apparently your nervous-system cells are not functioning properly. When they are not functioning properly, the results are also a malfunction of the motor function, sensory function and brain function. Schizophrenia, amnesia, and various types of paresthesias, could result. Megavitamin therapy is definitely worth a try. You might also check with a chiropractor. Sometimes a disturbed alignment in the first two cervicals, the atlas or axis, has caused amnesia, by cutting off circulation. An adjustment is a quick remedy.

Gynecomastia

Q. *I seem to have a case of gynecomastia. No matter how much I weigh or how much exercise I do, I always have breastlike fat deposits on my chest. At age 12 (I'm now 25) I had an operation for undescended testicles (2). Afterward my sexual maturation was very slow. Today I'm normal sexually. I'm happily married and a father. But I've found that unless I'm really careful about my diet and exercise a lot that I rapidly become flabby and soft. What can one do for this condition?*—S.B., Tulsa, Oklahoma.

A. Frankly, I do not know the answer to your problem. However I will do a little speculating. As you know, all individuals are neither pure male nor female in hormonal makeup. We all are some of both sexes. Each has his own balance. Some people are much more masculine than others and are physically developed accordingly. Others are much more feminine and are so built physically. The rest of us are somewhere in between.

You make me think that you are somewhere nearer the middle than most. Even though you are normal sexually and are a father, the development of the anatomy is less masculine than usual. As such you are then prone to develop some tendencies toward feminine type anatomic forms. So-called secondary sexual characteristics are more feminine than expected.

What to do about it is another thing. Theoretically, you could improve your masculinity by taking male sex hormones. But, this just does not seem to work. Other types of hormone therapy also seem to fail. Nutritionally, there is no answer known to me.

Liver Glycogen

Q. *My son and I have been diagnosed as having liver glycogen. I am asking your help in diet planning. Are* *there any foods especially good in treating this disease? I would like to begin nutritional therapy immediately.—* D.C., North Miami Beach, Fla.

A. Somehow you have your names crossed. Liver glycogen is the term used to designate the storage form of glucose in the liver. Glycogen is stored glucose which is the simple sugar which is the basis of sucrose or ordinary white sugar. There is, therefore, no disease called by the name liver glycogen.

Blood Levels

Q. *I would be thankful for any information on diet and/or supplement facts on high blood urea nitrogen—in cases where uric acid is normal but blood urea is high. There seem to be vast differing opinions: some say high protein, some low.*—H.H.N., New York, New York.

A. Blood uric acid and blood urea content are entirely different and cannot be considered together. Elevated blood urea, BUN, is caused by two conditions. The first is kidney damage and the second is the absorption of blood from the intestinal tract. The latter is called azotemia. Naturally, these two conditions are very different and must be treated differently. Treatment of uremia, the former, is the treatment of kidney conditions or nephritis. In my opinion, animal protein should be entirely eliminated during treatment. The increased animal protein puts an added strain on the kidneys so that healing cannot take place and the condition, in fact, is made worse. Vegetable protein is another story. Here the volume is not so important as is the quality. High quality protein is easily extracted from vegetable sources and can be used by the body. The vitamins and enzymes found in raw foods also aid in healing.

Smoking Addiction

Q. *Please! Is there anything that can be given to an addicted smoker to help him lose his taste for cigarettes? I take all of the minerals and vitamins and have tried to "ta-*

per off" with no success. I know that I am ruining my lungs.—B.A.L., Memphis, Tennessee.

A. To my knowledge, there is no nutritional aid to stop smoking. The only thing that seems to be of value is that when the patient is nutritionally well balanced, he has less desire to smoke.

High Uric Acid

Q. *Please give me all the information you have on high uric acid. Will a vegetable diet cure this condition?*—G.S., Garfield Heights, Ohio.

A. High uric acid in the system is a precursor of gout. I consider this to be evidence of liver failure. When there is liver failure, it means a total program in the largest sense of the word is needed.

There are so many ways to encourage liver cleansing that I really do not have the space to go into them here. Take large doses of the following materials for a long period of time and the liver will tend to correct itself. Eating raw organically raised liver or desiccated liver tablets is a good supportive measure for liver function. Garlic is a good cleanser. Even taking a clove of raw garlic each day may be enough to help but three times daily would be more sure. Many different regimens are available for your use.

Transurethal Resection

Q. *About one month ago I had a transurethal resection of prostate which was found benign, also a resection of bladder neck to correct a stricture. Recovery has been satisfactory—due in part, perhaps, to my knowledge of nutrition. Is there anything that I can specifically do in the area of nutrition which might be helpful to maintain better health in the case of a loss of the prostate gland?*—E.O., Arlington Heights, Ill.

A. A transurethal resection does not remove all the prostatic gland. At least a shell is retained. Therefore, it is important to do things which are good for prostatic tissue.

One major item is calcium and another is Vitamin F. Both are extra special insofar as the prostate is concerned as is raw prostate tissue extract.*

X Rays

Q. *I just finished a series of bladder and kidney X rays —15 or so. I just read Linda Clark's article on the dangers of X ray. What can I do to rebuild my system? Also, what causes a person to get poison ivy?*—Mrs. D.S., Tucker, Georgia.

A. Poison ivy, like poison oak, is an allergic response of the skin to the Rhus toxicodendron of the plant. Some people are less allergic to this poison than others.

There is no complete answer to the question of how to detoxify the body from radiation exposure. Vitamin C is foremost in my mind since it is a great detoxifier, and Vitamin E should be used to enhance the oxygen utilization of the system. Naturally, these vitamins are in addition to a strong nutritional program. Vitamin F has strong antiradiation effects. So does sodium alginate (found in health stores).

Other methods are mentioned in Linda Clark's book *Are You Radioactive? How to Protect Yourself.*

Various Deficiencies

Q. *I have all the symptoms of a pantothenic acid deficiency. I have white blotches on my legs, gray hair and I'm only 30. My hands and feet are always red and cold. I have low resistance. Two months ago I had strep throat and swollen glands in my neck and a few weeks ago I came down with the flu.*

How much pantothenic acid should I take a day and is there anything else I could take that would help this condition?

I take vitamins, eat sprouts, yogurt, lecithin and blackstrap molasses.

*See Product Information.

My gums are also starting to recede. What would be good for this? I would appreciate any help you could give me.—I.H., Redmond, Wash.

A. I would guess that you do not have just pantothenic acid deficiency, but probably multiple deficiencies. Get busy on a total program including all sorts of vitamins and minerals. Eat good natural foods, mostly raw.

Several Problems

Q. *Could you please tell me why, after eating anything, I always burp like a baby? I also break out on my face. I dry out the pimples with talcum powder, but they always come back. I do not have good elimination. Lately, I discovered a lump under my right breast. It hurts to the touch but is not visible. Do you have any suggestions for my many problems?*—K.S., Hamilton, Ontario, Canada.

A. The stem of your problem may well lie in the lack of hydrochloric acid. With this sort of lack, you are not able to digest your food properly; and this leads to gas and burping as a starter. Since you are not able to digest your foods properly, the rest of your body is subject to deterioration because of lack of proper nutrition.

To speculate about the lump under the breast is something else again. Any lump is considered cancerous until proven otherwise according to the orthodox medical experts. This is true especially around the breast. I would question your tumor as being cancerous because of the pain associated with it in such an early stage. Cancer is usually without pain. It probably represents a lymph node.

Various Problems

Q. *My mother, who is 62, is suffering great pain. Although she has had several tests in the past year, the doctors have left a big question mark as to whether she has Parkinson's disease. She is almost paralyzed on one side, and she has bursitis in the other shoulder, as well as neck pains, and her mouth is so sore she can hardly eat. She also has constipation. Do you have any suggestions for her various problems?*—J.C., Belleville, Ont.

A. Calcium is a physiological tranquilizer and analgesic especially where muscle spasm is involved. I really prefer the use of a naturally chelated substance.

Her paralysis is more difficult to remedy but one should try the use of raw brain tissue extract.* Sometimes the stimulation of the nerve cells themselves can cause an improvement in Parkinsonism. But, the nutritional treatment of nerve conditions is the least rewarding of all the types of nutritional problems. In other words, it is much easier and effective to cause improvement in liver or heart conditions than with nerve conditions.

The bursitis is an indication of shortage of chloride in the system. Hydrochloric acid can be a good source of chloride but I find that the salt preparation is better. (Salt in this case is not table salt or sodium chloride but whole sea salt.) Also, ammonium chloride is a good source of chloride.

Her sore mouth is indicative of severe B-complex deficiency. She needs the works here. The B complex can also be a benefit to the nerve function as well as to constipation.

*See Product Information.

34. Mouth and Throat

Saliva

Q. *What causes one's saliva to be stringy? Mine is at times.*—Mrs. E.L., San Diego, California.

A. Thick saliva is the result of too little water in the saliva. Too little water can be caused by not drinking enough water. You should consume enough water to produce 1½ quarts of urine per day. It could also be caused by disturbances in electrolyte (minerals) balance. Sodium, potassium, magnesium, calcium, manganese, iron, copper and zinc are some of the minerals which must be in balance in the body. You may produce too much saliva or not enough. It not enough, then it is usually too thick.

Mucous Membrane

Q. *For the past two months I have noticed a "gravel" sound in my throat (sounds like it involves the mucous membrane) and I wonder if I could be hurting my throat? After I sing now it feels a little raw and I really get upset. Could it be that I am not breathing correctly and putting too much effort on my throat? Also what would you suggest I do to cut down on mucus?*—G.W., Denver, Colorado.

A. Presumably you could be having difficulty in any part of the voice mechanism. It could be in the vocal cords or the voice box or the throat or the nose. I do not know where to start. A good examination would be in order.

Nutritionally, one should attack the problem in a manner wherein there are beneficial nutrients for this specific area. First there must be an adequacy of Vitamins A and C. Both are vital for mucous membrane integrity. Then there is Vitamin D and calcium. One must not forget the natural antihistamine liver hormone, *yakriton*.* From here one becomes more general. Since this part of the anatomy is a part of the body, one must support the whole body in the best manner as possible. Good liver function is a must if the nasal passages are to function properly.

Fenugreek as tea or in tablets is considered a good herbal treatment for mucus.

Sore Throat and Fever

Q. *Our 4½-year-old daughter is in good health, excepting that about three time a year she gets a sore throat and fever. The doctor wants to remove the tonsils, but we don't. Can you tell us what she is lacking in her diet?*—Mrs. B.F., Yorba Linda, Calif.

A. Giving a specific answer for this problem is difficult. It is much easier to say that your daughter can be helped by a good balanced nutritional regimen. First, there is Vitamin C. Adequate C helps to maintain proper resistance to infections. Likewise, Vitamin A. Both of these should be taken in large dosages. A third substance is raw lung tissue extract.* This substance can help to build up the integrity of the local tissue involved. In general, to help develop immunity, the use of raw thymus tissue extract* can aid the body in its ability to manufacture antibodies and thus throw off such chronic recurrent infections. Usually, nutritional deficiencies are multiple, not single, but this is at least a good way to begin correction of this particular problem.

Mucus

Q. *I am continually clearing small specks of mucus from my throat. I have had two cultures taken and both times the result was just the normal number of bacteria.*

I am positive there is an infection of some sort, but just

*See Product Information.

can't get an autogenous vaccine made. Do you have some suggestions?—W. W., Seattle, Wash.

A. If autogenous vaccine is what you want, I do not see why it cannot be done. Unless there is some very special complication, I do not understand why you cannot go to the nearest hospital laboratory to have the work done. On the other hand, if you wish to have a try at a nutritional method, I might suggest that you first load yourself with an abundance of good, natural Vitamin C. Plenty of A is needed too. Then you can take an enzymatic extract of raw thymus tissue.* This will help you to produce more effectively more immune bodies in the gamma globulin. This is a long-term type of treatment, but it is very valuable in many cases.

*See Product Information.

35. Muscular and Neuromuscular Diseases

Epilepsy

Q. *All of my life I have been very sick with epilepsy. As a child I would get very sick every time I ate apples or bananas and would get 15 to 20 seizures a day. I used to tell my doctor that I got sick from certain foods and he used to tell me that it was all in my head. Finally, my new neurologist asked if I had ever had a glucose tolerance test, and I said no. So they gave me one and found out that I had serious hypoglycemia, which naturally triggers the epilepsy. I have to take five Dilantin, four Mysoline and 4-5 Phenobarbitals a day (½ gr). They help to a certain point, but make me feel worn out and tired all of the time. Now my question is, do these drugs deplete your body of vitamins and minerals, and if so, which ones and how much would you suggest a person take with meals or in between meals? You have mentioned that a good detoxification is good for this. But there is something else I am afraid of because each time I eat something that gives me the runs, or have a case of intestinal flu with the runs, I get the seizures real bad. My blood sugar drops way down to nothing immediately. On top of all this I have gout, edema and Fordyce disease. My parotid glands hurt all the time and swell up by night time. Can this be a vitamin deficiency too?—V.P., Jr., Sacramento, California.*

A. My patients are almost all "other doctors' failures." Their stories are fantastic. All this has taught me a few pointers. The first one is to try to establish basic facts and not to be influenced too much by past experiences. Thus, my detoxification phase. After determining to the best of my ability the basic deficiencies in the system, I proceed to detoxify by using a very limited diet for a period of two weeks. This amounts to one or two preselected foods eight or more times daily, plus water. After the system is cleansed, I then begin to rebuild cells and structure. This takes a long time but can usually be accomplished. This is when I dig into the heavy megavitamin therapy of all types of vitamins and supplements and tissue extracts.

Thus, my answer to your problem: have a metabolic examination to determine your weaknesses and needs. Then go through a detoxification and, finally, a rebuilding program. It is not easy nor is it inexpensive, but it is rewarding. I have no idea as to the outcome of such a venture in your case. I do know that you can be benefitted, how much I cannot say. It is an individual problem. You are unique in your problems and in your solutions.

Epilepsy

Q. *I am troubled with epilepsy brought on by a strong emotional upset. When I live a normal life without any strong emotional problems, I seem to get along O.K., but when something comes along that bothers me, I have "blackout" spells, and because of this I am unable to obtain a driver's license in this state.*

Any suggestions will be very gratefully received.— H. J. P., Portland, Ore.

A. Epilepsy is a condition wherein the brain emits abnormal impulses, particularly motor impulses, which cause the body to react in an overactive manner, even to the extent of stimulating a convulsion. The degree of the reaction is called *petit mal* or *grand mal*, ranging from the very minor and minute phase to the major convulsion. The various causes of this illness can be types of brain damage or scar tissue therein. Sometimes there is an obvious metabolic disturbance in the patient. Mostly, the diagnosis is: "Epilepsy, cause unknown."

In my experience, I have found that a great many of the "unknown" cases can be traced to abnormal metabolic utilization of sugar in the system, a condition known as low blood sugar, or hypoglycemia. The diagnosis is made by the proper interpretation of the five-hour glucose tolerance test. If this diagnosis can be made, then the full program for the treatment of hypoglycemia should be instituted at once. This is a whole program and cannot be summarized in terms like: "Eat no sugar" or "Eat a diet high in protein," or "When you feel poorly, just eat a candy bar." These are some of the types of advice still being offered to patients today. In my opinion such advice (especially the latter type) just contributes to a worsening of the problem. It represents gross ignorance of the problem.

In my estimation, a full dietary program must be planned. There must be a full food supplemental program to provide the patient with all his particular needs as well as the generalized needs. There should also be a definite program of adrenocortical support, with the aim of correcting the metabolic problem therein. Pancreatic, hepatic, thyroid and pituitary support are critical areas to be considered in total therapy.

When this sort of a program is instituted, one suddenly finds that he can treat epilepsy without using the anticonvulsive drugs to a very great extent.

Another method of treatment that should be mentioned here is the use of large doses of magnesium. Some experts say that epilepsy can be cured by dosages of magnesium in the range of 450 milligrams per day. Also, the administration of Vitamin B-6 can sometimes help epileptic seizures to cease. Vitamin B-2 should also be added to insure proper nerve function. Conditions such as idiopathic epilepsy are in reality systemic diseases which require total body metabolic support for proper management.

Muscular Dystrophy

Q. *A friend of mine has a pretty bad case of muscular dystrophy. He has been everywhere and seems to find no help. As I am a firm believer in vitamins, minerals and the like—I can't help but believe that this ailment is brought on by some nutritional deficiency. Can you offer any suggestions?*—M. B., Middlebury, Indiana.

A. Muscular dystrophy is a condition arising from defective or faulty nutrition of the muscles. It usually affects the muscles of the shoulder girdle first and the muscles become enlarged, then atrophy later.

However, it is not the usual malnutrition which causes

the problem as such. It is some sort of defect which causes malnutrition of the individual muscle cells.

Just how much of this is inherent enzymatic defect and how much is nutritional in the usual sense of the word I do not know. However, just because we do not know, does not mean that we do not try to support the muscle tissue. All nutrients are essential for normal bodily function. With muscles we can emphasize protein, calcium, magnesium, potassium, sodium, manganese, iron, trace minerals, Vitamins A, B, C, D, E, F, fatty acids, etc. *All nutrients are essential*. Raw muscle tissue extract* can be of assistance for enhancement of normalcy. RNA makes individual cells work better. All these can be used to support muscle metabolism and normal function.

Of course, one must be able to digest these various nutrients. For this one needs hydrochloric acid, pepsin, bile salts and pancreatic enzymes. All are a part of the total picture. Every patient is unique and must be handled as a separate entity and demands the complete metabolic analysis to determine his particular needs.

Recently a 10:1 wheat germ oil concentrate has been developed by Viobin Corporation. This preparation contains a neuromuscular factor and so states on the label. Unfortunately, large doses of this expensive substance are needed for control of neuromuscular diseases. Also, it is a prolonged effort.

Difficulty Swallowing

Q. I have a problem that I have never seen discussed. It is difficulty in swallowing. I have told this to my doctor during one of my yearly physicals, but he did not say anything nor recommend anything; nevertheless it bothers me very much. Perhaps it is some deficiency of nutrients or minerals.

Whenever I try to swallow some vitamins, they get lodged in my throat. I quickly take a bit of whatever is handiest, banana, potato or even bread. While I am chewing the pill works its way up or, if it stays put, I swal-

*See Product Information.

low whatever I am eating to help get it down. Then the food goes down, but not the pill.—R.A., Pleasant Garden, N.C.

A. Difficulty in swallowing makes me think of some sort of paralysis of the swallowing muscles. This could be due to polio or some such. It could also be due to chemical poisoning. At the meeting place of the nerves and muscles, the synapse, the nerve impulse spreads to the muscle and thus a contraction will result. The administration of choline and pantothenic acid may help. It will strengthen the weakened muscles so that they contract appropriately. About 1000 mg of both items is needed per day, but build up the dosage slowly because the body may not be able to tolerate sudden input of such large doses.

The 10:1 wheat germ oil concentrate could strengthen these muscles, too.

Incidentally, a way to get pills down is to have a mouthful of food all chewed and ready to swallow. Toss in a few pills, mix with the tongue and swallow. When one needs to take lots of pills, this is a way to lessen the chore.

Multiple Sclerosis

Q. *I have multiple sclerosis and have had it for at least 20 years. There are many disturbing side-symptoms: cold hands and feet, nausea, muscle pain and spasms, and ringing in my right ear, which trouble me.*

I have gone to doctors and more doctors, but no answers. The only thing I found out was that I have hypoglycemia (low blood sugar), but I still believe there is something that can be done for me. I believe anything that is wrong with me is my fault and something can be done for it and I also believe that what we eat and drink has a lot to do with it.

I will tell you something I did. Maybe you will think I should go to a psychiatrist, but I am still here. I read about Vitamin E and the reports I read were all so good, I started to take it on my own; my first mistake. I started 200 IU 3 times a day and felt wonderful. I did that for a week then tried 400 IU three times a day for another week and felt so good. Walking improved and everything.

*Then I figured, why not double that amount? So I did, 800
IU three times a day and still felt good. I thought I had
my multiple sclerosis whipped, so I figured—one more
jump and I've got it made, so here goes: 1,600 IU three
times a day. In two days I was in the hospital. I thought I
had a heart attack, but the doctors told me no. My blood
pressure was 170 over 80. I just stayed in the hospital 3
days and was released. I can't take Vitamin E anymore.
When I do, I think I am having a heart attack. I am 48
years old, 5 feet 8½ and weight 160 lbs., but want to
weigh 150 so I am cutting all food in half. I went from
180 lbs. to 160 lbs. in six months. Now my weight drop is
slowing to about 2-3 lbs. a month. Is there any diet you
could suggest?—F.H.K.*

A. Multiple sclerosis is a neurological disease where
there is wasting away of muscular tissue because of the
failure of the integrity of the nerve tissue. In my estimation, the nerve tissue is deteriorated because of nutritional
imbalances. The deterioration in the nerve tissue does not
occur in one place nor in a single nerve system but, rather,
occurs in an irregular, sporadic manner. There is no pattern to the deterioration. It is a disease where there may
be short periods of remission but there is usually a gradual
but steady deterioration in function.

Your experience with Vitamin E is very interesting.
You did not mention what brand of E you were taking so
I cannot comment. However, there is all the difference in
the world between brands. I believe in that derived from
the so-called natural sources, including the four types of
tocopherols and containing all the naturally occurring
synergistic micronutrients. This is a must. You can get into
severe difficulty otherwise. Do not be so hasty in trying to
find your level of dosage. You should not increase the
daily dosage for at least a couple of weeks; even a month
is more reasonable. Also do not get too anxious to find the
proper end point. Feel your way slowly. Allow for cumu-
lative effects of the dosage which has already been taken.
Take your time. You have had the condition for 20 years
and another couple of months will not make that much
difference now.

You cannot correct basic problems if you do not supply

the body the building blocks with which to do the repairing.

I cannot possibly prescribe a diet for you without knowing more about you. A complete metabolic analysis is necessary before such things can even be considered. And keep praying!

Multiple Sclerosis

Q. *What is being done for multiple sclerosis in this country?*—D. K., Bronx, New York.

A. Multiple sclerosis is a condition of the nerve tissues where certain cells are killed. When killed, they no longer function, so there is a defect in the total nervous system. In my opinion, the effect of poor nutritional intake plus the increased intake of chemicals or nonfoods are the main factors. What can be done when the condition has developed? Frankly, it is the same nutritional approach necessary to supply *all* the basic nutrients to the body. The supply must be in abundance, not just minimal. The mineral intake must be complete and abundant, too.

It is my impression that multiple sclerosis is in the early stages when the patient may have certain polyneuritic complaints. These may include such things as slurred speech, labile temper, double vision, transient pruritis or itching of the skin, transient weaknesses even as noted after the "flu," disturbed reflex tests on examination, etc. Any sort of neurological abnormality can be considered to be the early stages of multiple sclerosis. I can say that I have been able to nip the process in the bud in several cases, before the death of the nerve cells. As long as the nerves are still alive, they can be improved. No improvement is possible, however, after the cells are dead.

Interestingly, the use of large and prolonged doses of RNA can be of value. It may even seem as if some cells are brought back to life. In one case, the patient had a very severe cerebral hemorrhage involving the basilar artery. This is usually a fatal condition, but he did not die. He was, however, paralyzed from the neck down. He was started on a total nutritional program administered by stomach tube, since he could not swallow. Among other things, he was given large doses of RNA. This program was continued for 13 months. At the end of this time, he was able to move quite well with only a slight weakness of the right arm. He was even able to go to work. Usually, patients who have had cerebral accidents think about past events, even childhood memories. This man did not do so. In fact, he was making plans for future improvements. Unfortunately, he became careless in his continuing to consume large doses of RNA which led to a recurrence of his cerebral accident, from which he succumbed. The point is, however, he did survive the first time and apparently revitalized dead nerve tissue. Naturally, one case does not prove a point, but it may plant some seeds.

Amyotrophic Lateral Sclerosis

Q. *What is the difference between amyotrophic lateral sclerosis and multiple sclerosis?*—B. H., Troy, New York.

A. I believe the cause of amyotrophic lateral sclerosis is no different from that of multiple sclerosis. The main difference is the location of the lesions.

Myasthenia Gravis

Q. *I am inquiring about your treatment of myasthenia gravis. I have suffered from this disease for three years and am being treated with Mesthinon by a neurologist. This drug merely relieves the symptoms (somewhat) but it certainly does not cure it. For the past five weeks I have been under a complete nutritional program by another doctor. However, I have felt worse since being on this complete program than when I was on my own more haphazard one. It is very puzzling to me and to my doctor who knows very little about the disease. The weakness normally experienced with the disease has increased to where I can hardly move my arms or eat, but when the supplements are stopped for a day the mobility returns. Nutritionally, I have improved—my blood pressure at the start was 88/50 and now is 105/65, plus slight improvements in the other vitamin deficiencies. Do you have any suggestions for my problem?*—G. W., Westerly, R.I.

A. The first thing to understand is why clinical symptoms get worse when the correct things are given. Picture it this way: the body is constantly trying to obtain harmony or balance. When there is disease present, this interferes with the balance. When the correct treatment is used, the abnormality may begin to be corrected, but the balance is still decidedly out of kilter. Thus, even if the patient is improving, the clinical symptoms may be getting worse. Improvement in clinical symptoms may not be forthcoming until the abnormality in levels of nutrients is corrected. Thus, a patient may appear to get worse before getting better.

What nutritional items you need is a question. You need them all in very optimal amounts. You are probably vitamin dependent, which is saying that you probably need large dosages of supplements and that these dosages must be continued for long periods of time, even life. You need them all, even choline and manganese. I would lean heavily on raw heart tissue extract* as a means of stimulating the muscle. Naturally, there must be support in the form of all vitamins, minerals, enzymes, hormones, etc. in abundance. In some situations, one may need ten pills per day but if only eight are taken, the results may not be forthcoming because the need is not satisfied.

Calcium should be one of your most urgent needs. When taking calcium, one must adjust it against phosphorus, against magnesium, against sodium, potassium, etc. as well as against the parathyroid hormone. And do not forget Vitamin D. It is essential for proper calcium metabolism. Finally, liquid lecithin has reportedly helped myasthenia gravis.

Myasthenia Gravis

Q. *Can you give me some information about myasthenia gravis? I have a very dear friend who has this disease and I would like to know if there is anything that can be done.*—Mrs. G. B., Hartford, Conn.

A. Myasthenia gravis is no different than any other disease entity when spoken of nutritionally. This means that it is the patient and not the condition which needs treat-

*See Product Information.

ment. The complete metabolic analysis is of the utmost importance. When individual differences are determined, then a more specific muscle-favoring program can be set up. I would certainly give raw muscle tissue extract* and raw heart tissue. Beyond this, I would add pantothenic acid and choline 1000 mgm each per day for good myoneural function. Lecithin has also proved helpful on occasion.

Myasthenia Gravis

Q. *It has recently been diagnosed that my 11-year-old daughter has myasthenia gravis. We are advised there is no cure for this disease. The symptoms began about six months ago in the form of nasal speech and lack of control of lip muscles (cannot say "stirring" or "judges" very well), droopy eyes, tires easily, irritable, temperamental, and occasional dizziness.*

Recently I have become frightfully aware that the nutrition of my family has not been given the proper attention. We have always had to watch our pennies to make ends meet, and therefore I rarely purchased fresh fruit. All of our vegetables were canned or frozen, except we did have tossed salads frequently, the breads were white with preservatives, and fruit juices were canned and more of a drink than a juice.

We have now made a new start, but I wonder if our eating habits over the last 11 years contributed to my daughter's illness. She had vitamins as a baby up until she was about four years old. Two weeks ago, I started her on some high potency C/B-Complex vitamins with digestive enzymes, one capsule a day, and also a grocery store variety of daily multiple vitamins with iron. She is also taking a drug called Mesthinon, one or two a day as needed, which acts as a temporary stimulant to her muscles.

She has always been a happy, energetic, and adorable child, the oldest of three children, and a sheer delight to her father and me. It breaks our hearts to see what is happening to her. The doctors have suggested having her thymus gland removed, should she get any worse, as a possible deterrent to this disease. However, they frankly say

*See Product Information.

they do not know if it will have any effect or not, as there are no medical facts on what the thymus gland really does past the age of seven.

Is there anything that I might try that you could suggest to help my little girl? We have nothing to lose by trying, and everything to gain.

A. Myasthenia gravis is a degenerative muscular disease characterized by the inability to make the muscles work properly both in the sense of strength and in the sense of repeated or sustained action. In the first sense, there is some weakness, and in the latter sense, there is a shortening of the contraction time before exhaustion of the muscle occurs. It also means that there is some inability to repeat contractions in speedy series without exhaustion and utter inability to do so sets in. Thus there are some characteristic findings, as mentioned in the letter, such as speech and swallowing difficulties.

There is no known cause, and consequently, no known orthodox remedy for this condition.

However, from the nutritional viewpoint, this is not the time to give up and not try to evoke *some* sort of response. Nutritionally, we are always searching for some means of strengthening the defenses of the body against whatever adverse force is present. In this case, we are looking for something to strengthen the function of the muscles. In my experience, the use of raw muscle tissue extract* is of some value. Vitamin E aids in the circulation to the area as well as enhancing the utilization of oxygen once it gets to the tissue. That is to say that the internal respiration is implemented. Vitamin C is always good to aid in the bolstering of the general defensive mechanisms of the body, mainly by enhancing the adrenal cortical function. Anything that will aid in the liver's job of removing waste products from the system would be of value in aiding the defensive mechanisms. Many things can be done to stimulate liver action. Various mechanisms have been mentioned in this column on various occasions. Read about the case of myasthenia gravis which responded to lecithin, described in Linda Clark's paperback book *Secrets of Health and Beauty.* Lecithin has been found helpful.

*See Product Information.

As with other so-called hopeless situations, I have found personally that a good serious attempt to alter the favorable factors can sometimes result in miracles. This is not to say that there is a cure for myasthenia gravis, but proper food supplements will give results many times where the wrong ones will not.

Myositis

Q. *My condition was diagnosed as myositis. I have been to many doctors, even to a well-known clinic and spent lots of money, all to no avail. One doctor gave me injections of B-12 which were supposed to do the trick, but they didn't. Another doctor said there are many kinds of myositis and he would have to know which one I had before he could treat me. I can't seem to find out exactly what it is, and what is the cause, but I would appreciate so much if someone could help me with this problem.*

I am 62 years of age and in need of exercise, but any I try causes muscular soreness. My muscles seem to have shortened and stretching them causes a lot of pain.—A.J. Gerard, Tulsa, Oklahoma.

A. Myositis is an inflammatory condition involving the muscles. It is probably due to a protein loss. Protein loss can be caused by several different things. First, the insufficient intake of protein or a poor quality intake. Or, if the intake is adequate, there may be a problem in the digestion of the protein. Even then, the digested elements or amino acids, may not be utilized for one reason or another. Finally, the excretion of the waste products may be malfunctioning, which could cause the loss of protein from the system.

The first thing I would start you on would be hydrochloric acid in the form of betaine hydrochloride. This should be combined with pepsin and should be taken after or late in the meal. Larger dosages should be taken when the meal is high in protein. A high protein diet can do nothing in itself unless it is digested.

Another point that must be considered here is the sufficiency of Vitamin E. I prefer the natural E, d-alpha tocopherol. Take large dosages, say 800 mg per day. If this is not enough to do the job, the dosage can go as high as 1600 mg, but should be raised to that level slowly. See the book *Vitamin E for Ailing and Healthy Hearts,* by Wilfrid E. Shute, M.D.

Amyotrophic Lateral Sclerosis

Q. *If the nerves in the spine have deteriorated, with scars; and the muscles, in turn, have shrunk (the doctor calls it amyotrophic lateral sclerosis); and the voice has become quavery, what program would be most beneficial to cure, or at least arrest, the condition? There is also presence of angina and low blood sugar. The patient takes no drugs whatsoever.*—O.L., Chicago, Ill.

A. By the time you have reached the stage of deterioration of the muscles, it is very late in the game. To the best of my knowledge, dead cells do not return to life. Death of a cell is permanent and if enough cells are dead, you have extreme problems. The best that one can hope to accomplish in such a condition is to halt the progress of degeneration. To do this requires an all-out effort for a long period of time. Even this can be less than satisfactory.

By an all-out effort, I mean that the entire metabolic status of the body must be evaluated by physical histories, functional tests, and analytic laboratory tests of the blood and urine. When a physician accumulates such a complete evaluation of the patient, he can begin to formulate a program designed to strengthen tissues which are not already destroyed. All tips and clues found from such an evaluation should be pursued and definite steps should be taken to make the appropriate correction.

The angina and low blood sugar are incidental to the total condition, but they are very important. Angina concerns a vital organ, the heart, and thus can become a problem way out of proportion to the degree of involvement. That is to say that a small lesion in the heart could become a vital issue under the wrong circumstances. Low blood sugar is a problem which may not cause primary problems itself, but it certainly does contribute to the magnitude of many other problems including amyotrophic lateral sclerosis and angina. When the sugar level is low, many other things are much more likely to happen than if the blood sugar level is normal.

Incidentally, amyotrophic lateral sclerosis involves the degeneration of the nerve cells located in the lateral column of the spinal cord. These cells are the ones primarily associated with the motor functions of the muscles. They do not, for instance, have anything to do with sensation; they are motor nerves. That is why the muscles deteriorate; no nerve impulses get to the muscles through the dead nerve cells, so the muscles themselves can also eventually atrophy.

Amyotrophic Lateral Sclerosis

Q. *A good friend of mine is afflicted with amyotrophic lateral sclerosis. What can nutrition do for her?*—G.B., West Hartford, Connecticut.

A. Amyotrophic lateral sclerosis is a result of nutritional deficiency like almost all other degenerative diseases. I believe that the basic weakness which allows most diseases to develop is nutritional deficiency. From then, there are many different factors which contribute to the breakdown of the tissues. A very important point to remember is that there is always a point of no return. In other words, the deterioration may progress to a point where it can no longer be corrected. When tissue is dead, it is dead. This is particularly true with nerve tissue. However, in the same breath, I will say that one never knows when a cell is just severely insulted or whether it is dead. If it is the former, then some kinds of therapy can be of assistance. By this I mean, good nutrition can be beneficial. Like a sprained ankle—not all the cells are involved but there is much swelling involving many cells.

There are no specifics in nutritional therapy for this disturbance, just the all-round good basic nutritional formula: Plenty of all the nutrients, at appropriate intervals and for a long enough period of time. If you are on the right track, the results should be forthcoming. Remember this, each and every one of us has his own specific dosages needed for proper functioning of his own body. Every person is unique and needs particular balances to make his individual metabolism function properly. This is why one particular substance could certainly cure a special situation in one person but not do any such thing for another. It is like a giant jigsaw puzzle: There is always a last piece. So there is always the last addition to the nutritional program which may seem like it is the magic item and causes a cure overnight.

Antimetabolites

Q. *What can you tell me about L-Dopa, Dispisal and Valium? I read that multivitamins and minerals should not be taken with L-Dopa. Can you tell me why?*—A.H., Vancouver, Washington.

A. You have opened the Pandora's Box. However, I am not going to say more than that these drugs, as are all drugs, are antimetabolites. This means they block normal metabolic processes in one manner or another. This is the basic difference between vitamins and drugs. Drugs never cure anything and neither do vitamins. The cure comes from within the body. The body itself makes the cure as it regains normal function. Vitamins tend to aid and abet normal function while drugs tend to further assist deterioration but do not accomplish balance so that there is general improvement even if the body is not functioning normally.

L-Dopa and Dispisal are kinds of antitremor drugs. Valium is a tranquilizer. All work on the central nervous system. All are antimetabolites of sorts. All work contrary to vitamins and often produce side effects.

Parkinson's Disease

Q. *My husband has been a victim of Parkinson's disease for nearly eight years. His case is a rare one accompanied by severe pain. For two years he has been on L-Dopa, which has helped the tremor, but the pain seems increasingly more severe. We have been informed by his doctor not to give him Vitamin B-6 (pyridoxine) because of its* *conflict with L-Dopa. He does take a special vitamin made by the company which makes the drug, and also calcium, magnesium and pantothenic acid. Because of his constant pain, we are wondering what your opinion would be in regard to discontinuing the L-Dopa and putting him on a heavy vitamin program?*—M.A., Idaho Falls, Idaho.

A. I have no real answer for nerve disease problems such as Parkinsonism. The best I can say is that if the nerve cells are not already dead, they can be rescued, but that, if they are dead, that is that! Unfortunately, one cannot tell if the cells are already dead or just insulted without a good clinical trial of the nutritional methods. Sometimes one is very pleasantly surprised, while the reverse is true, too.

Up to this point, I have not heard that Vitamin B-6 interferes with L-Dopa therapy. The vitamins that you mention as manufactured by the company involved are probably synthetics. This is an educated guess.

In my limited experience with L-Dopa, it appears that it is not the great solution to the problem as it has been touted. Many times the exact symptoms it is used to treat, i.e., the tremor, are made worse after a short period of benefit. In fact, the deterioration as a result of the L-Dopa can be permanent. Thus, I do not use it in my practice.

As stated above, the nutritional approach is sometimes beneficial and sometimes without noticeable effect. One does not know until it is tried.

Parkinson's Disease

Q. *What causes Parkinson's disease? Is there anything one can do healthwise to stem its progress? My sister has it and the medication prescribed makes her dizzy and miserable although it did help a little.*—L.M.J., Peidmont, California.

A. Parkinson's disease, or paralysis agitans, is classified as a disease of later life, progressive in character and marked by masklike facies, a characteristic tremor of resting muscles, a slowing of voluntary movements, a hurried gait, peculiar posture, and weakness of the muscles. There may be sweating and feelings of heat. The cause of the disease is a deterioration of nerve tissue, especially that of the cerebellum. What causes the deterioration of the nerve tissue is another story. One can say that there may be a hardening of the arteries to that specific area which results in insult and finally death to the nerve tissues involved. Once tissue is dead, it cannot be revived. Nerve tissue is very susceptible to the effects of lack of oxygen as compared with muscle tissue, for instance. Thus, if the tissue is dead, the answer is that nothing can be done. If it is only insulted, then there may be some sort of answer if the oxygen supply can be increased to the tissue at once. The use of Vitamin E is a good starter. It works amazingly well most of the time. Another thing that improves the circulation is the use of vitamin B-2. Anything that can begin to cause the arteries to soften a bit is of value. Here I suggest the use of lecithin. Dosages of this must be accompanied by calcium if it is given over a period of time. Raw nerve tissue extract* can be used to great advantage to try to normalize the function of the nerve tissue. All of these added together with a basic liver detoxification program can be a good nutritional approach to the problem. However, the results to be obtained by this method of therapy are not visible for a considerable period of time. The response of nerve tissue to therapy seems to be the slowest of all the tissues in the body. In regard to diseases of the nerve tissues, I consider that if the condition is just prevented from getting worse it is a successful program.

Parkinson's Disease

Q. *My husband, 63, has had Parkinson's disease for two years and seems to be getting worse. This disease is affecting the mental powers more than the motor functions. Is there any help for him at this stage, if only to arrest the condition? We are now taking B-6, Vitamin E and lecithin which I realize should have been used years ago. Are there any suggested dosages?*—Mrs. B.W., Wescoesville, Pennslyvania.

A. Parkinson's disease is a condition involving the brain cells. It is one which results, in extreme situations, in intensive tremor of the hands and arms. There are several drugs used to control this condition. Some are helped, whereas others are made worse by these medications. Nutritionally, there is little to offer.

Brain cells respond to therapy much more slowly than do the other tissues of the body. I would give those elements which have a particular use in the brain. Lecithin, Vitamin B complex, B-6, natural carbohydrates (raw fruits), calcium and magnesium are some of the important ones to remember as a start. Large doses of these items are quite important for normal brain function. There is no point in giving just a few of these items and then waiting to see results. All should be taken simultaneously in large and prolonged dosage.

Sore Muscles

Q. *I work for a large construction company. Many of the men complain of sore muscles or nerves in arms. No soreness in joints. Do you have any information as to a possible cause? The only thing I can find that may apply is the improper oxidation of carbohydrates caused by a deficiency of Vitamin B complex. Do you have any other information that might apply?*—O.A.M., Lincoln, Nebraska.

A. This is a most unusual problem. The first thing that occurs to me is that there is some sort of chemical in the environment which can cause such a condition. I do not know of such a thing offhand, but you may investigate. This reaction could be possible from exposure to the radiation emitted by microwave towers. If there is one in the vicinity, this could be the answer.

Some suggestions as to treatment are to be sure that there is adequate lecithin intake. I would suggest the liquid form, one teaspoonful three times daily. Moisten your mouth and/or the spoon with grapefruit juice first and then the lecithin will not stick so easily. Be sure that you have an adequacy of calcium, too. The increase in lecithin, which is a phospholipid, will deplete the calcium. I find I get good results with raw bone meal.

Your suggestion of natural B complex is good. If this proves to be a contamination of radiation from the microwave towers or some such, I would appreciate knowing this. In fact, if any of the readers know of anything positive in this vein, please let us know.

High calcium intake can be of value in muscular distress.

36. Nervous Ailments

Nervous Condition

Q. *Three doctors tell me my trouble is a nervous condition. It started gradually. My voice was the first to be affected, then my right arm started to jerk. I can't write with it at all. Some time later my left arm began to be affected the same way. The only way I can write with my left hand is to put the pencil between my first and second fingers and brace with my last three fingers. I have plenty of strength; it is the tedious things that cause the most trouble.*

After I started doing yoga exercises, I noticed a heavy white coating on my tongue every morning. It does not cause a bad taste. I scrape off an amount equal to the size of a lima bean every morning. Could the tensing of the nerves cause this?

My skin is so dry that my lips have dead skin on them most of the time, and my legs from the knees down look like crinkled crepe. My doctor tells me I am not absorbing some vitamin, but he doesn't tell me what to do.—Mrs. C.F.C., Jacksonville, Fla.

A. You are grossly toxic and need a detoxification program at once. You show evidence of neurological malfunction. You also show evidence of poor digestion. If the digestive problem is not solved, there will be a continuance of the wrong digestive elements getting into the system from the intestines and this, in turn, will further decrease the digestive activity.

Where to start in your case is the big problem. You need so much so soon. My approach would be to start you on a thorough liver detoxification program. Next, I would start to rebuild your digestive function. Both of these programs can be carried on simultaneously.

One of the most valuable individual items that I have

found in such instances is the use of hydrochloric acid. If the digestion in the stomach is not correct, due to the shortage or absence of hydrochloric acid, then all the rest of the digestive function is not correct. You then absorb the wrong substances supposed to be in the food.

Another way to begin to make your body function properly is to consume only one type of raw food, such as carrot juice, or grapes, etc. You could even accomplish this by eating only a raw diet, but in this case you should not eat fruits and vegetables at the same meal. For instance, you could consume fruits in the morning and evening and vegetables only at noon.

Along with these suggestions, it is wise not to consume too much food. If you eat more than the body can digest, you are only adding to your problem, even though you are eating only raw foods. Wtih a strict raw diet, you should begin to see your body improving in short order.

Later, when your body is in much better condition, you will find that meat is necessary to continue to provide the energy you need. Here again, the amount you require is probably much less than the amount that you think you should consume.

Naturally, during this whole program, you must be sure to consume all the vitamin supplements needed, as well as the minerals.

Neuritis?

Q. *I am now 44 years young, 5' 5" tall and weigh 125 lbs. Recently I awoke with a sore right knee. Soon it was "very tight" and swollen and the inner portion of my whole right leg was partially numb from my crotch to my toes. I went to a chiropractor for adjustment. The tightness around my knee receded until walking down the hall one evening, I had a short breath-taking pain in my right knee and it tightened again. That was the only pain. Use of the leg muscles was not apparently secure that way. I gave up the chiropractor after 2½ months, since there was no apparent improvement from treatments and no satisfying explanations were forthcoming. Now, after five months, I still have some numbness in the front part of my right foot and toes. It is improving "slowly." I would like to know if this partial numbness is actually caused only by a pinched nerve in the spinal column, or could there be a nutritional problem—a deficiency of a certain vitamin or mineral?*—M.W., Tahoe City, California.

A. The numbness which you mention in the extremities is quite likely to be secondary to neuritis. This neuritis can be mechanical in the sense that there is bone and joint pressure on a nerve as you suggested, and which the chiropractor was able to help. This is a very real problem and can be alleviated by manipulation most of the time. However, manipulation cannot reach biochemical problems. In your case, I suspect that you suffer from a deficiency of B-6 (pyridoxine). I usually use this vitamin in combination with B-3. You may also suffer from a deficiency of Vitamin E. This can cause neurologic disturbances.

Neuritis

Q. *I am hoping that you will be able to tell me what might relieve the pain of neuritis in my back.*—F.H.B., Peoria Heights, Illinois.

A. Neuritis, wherever it occurs, is the same. It is an inflammation of the nerve sheath so that the whole nerve is irritated. This irritation results in pain or weakness if the nerve is sensory or motor, respectively.

The major substance to correct neuritis is Vitamin B complex. This should be given in gigantic doses over as long a period as necessary to relieve the nerve irritation. One can take large doses of Vitamin C also. Calcium is a natural tranquilizer along with magnesium and you have the major basics for nerve function.

For temporary relief of pain, a little trick that doctors can use is ethyl chloride as a local spray. Locate the area next to the spinal column where there is a maximum tenderness. Aim the spray of the ethyl chloride next to the spinal crests and freeze a strip of skin about one-half inch in width for a distance of two or three vertebral spaces. This blocks the peripheral reflex cycle and interrupts the pain pattern. One treatment may give almost permanent relief. If not so lucky, the relief may only last a day or so.

Meanwhile step up your intake of the B complex in brewer's yeast powder and desiccated liver tablets.

Neuritis Sciatica

Q. *I have a neuritis sciatica and wonder what vitamins are the best and in what quantity. I have been to many types of doctors over the years and had X ray and muscle relaxant pills by the hundreds. My trouble is mostly in my right thigh and I only feel it when I cross my legs and also when driving—I use my left foot on the gas pedal so that I do not put any pressure on my bad leg. I am 51 and in pretty good health otherwise.*—Mr. J.T., No. Attleboro, Massachusetts.

A. Neuritis sciatica simply means that the sciatic nerve that goes into the leg is irritated and/or inflamed. It is just the same as neuritis in any other part of your anatomy. The symptomatic results can be quite variable due to the tissue involved, but this is all secondary to the nerve damage in the first place.

The therapeutic approach would be to do any and everything which would lessen the load carried by the nerves. First, would be to take large doses of B complex. Natural B-vitamin foods like brewer's yeast and liver should be supplemented by large doses of the separate factors like thiamin, niacin, pyridoxine, folic acid, B-12, etc. These all have a very beneficial effect on nerves. Next, the diet should be high in available protein. This point is well covered in liver and yeast therapy but other forms of protein can be included. Fish and other sea food are good sources. Sprouted grains and seeds are relatively high in protein of high quality and can be used. Next, one should insure adequate intake of minerals. Calcium and magnesium are the chief minerals used by nerve tissue. Of course there must be a balance of all the minerals as well as the vitamins and other food supplements.

Tissue supplements like raw brain and nerve tissue extracts* can also be of great assistance in such cases.

A chiropractor can usually relieve sciatics within

*See Product Information.

minutes, if it is due to a lack of alignment in the vertebrae, a common cause, or a dislocated sacroiliac joint.

Nervousness

Q. *I am nervous. I haven't taken any nerve pills for
about nine months and I hope I do not have to in the future. Do you know of any foods or diet or vitamin pills I
could take to help my nervousness?*—J.K., Indianapolis,
Ind.

A. One of the characteristics of nervousness is tension
of muscles. It is well known that calcium deficiencies can
cause spasms in the muscles. Therefore, it is logical to
conclude that calcium therapy can aid in some cases of
nervousness. I prefer to use raw bone meal that contains
magnesium*.

Another condition which commonly exists with nervousness is irritability of the nerves. By this I mean that the
actual anatomical nerve cell is more subject to stimulation
by the biochemical stimuli than normally. If this is the
case, then the use of certain members of the B-complex
group should be of value in treatment. This proves to be
the situation because Vitamins B-3 and B-6 both act in this
manner. Of course, these factors should be balanced with
the other members of the B complex. I do not believe in
the separate massive dosages of individual vitamin factors,
for the following reasons:

(1). Individual vitamin factors are synthetic or so completely purified from natural sources that there is no real
difference between them and the synthetics.

(2). Large dosages of single vitamin factors do not balance the other factors; they only add to the imbalance.
There may be good results at first, but this is only temporary. All synergistic micronutrients are necessary.

Nerve Function Disturbance

Q. *My wife has developed a very, very acute sense of
smell. No one can possibly believe the limits and restric-*

*See Product Information.

*tions it puts on her; and to add to the misery, most all
types of chemicals such as sprays, paints and even some
flowers and many other things too numerous to mention
give her headaches, burning of the mucous membranes,
nose, throat, stomach, and the lungs. She also has a sensitivity to many drugs and vitamins. Do you have any suggestions as to what she might do to alleviate this problem?
—J.M., Pa.*

A. This acuteness of smell is a situation brought on by
disturbance in nerve function. It is a type of neuritis.
Some of the things which should be of value are much Vitamin B complex. It would also be wise to take raw nerve
tissue extract* and a good supply of minerals, especially
calcium and magnesium.

Dead Nerve Cells

Q. *Our 18-year-old son received a broken neck resulting
in immediate paralysis from the neck down. The doctors
at the rehabilitation center believe it was a contusion frac-
ture of C-5 with a badly bruised spinal cord, but no
severance. He spent 10 weeks there and we brought him
home because their food was not of the type to promote
healing and recovery. We have been giving him many vitamins and minerals in megavitamin doses plus yogurt daily
to counteract the effects of oral antibiotics which caused
allergy reactions. He was also given electrical therapy
treatments twice weekly to keep the nerve pathways alive.
Is there any way to reestablish the nerve pathways through
the injured areas since his reflexes are still good?*—C.D.,
Flagstaff, Arizona.

A. You ask a question which is very difficult to answer.
When the nerve cells are dead, nothing will bring them
back to life. If the nerve cells are just insulted, then they
can be reactivated if the cause of the insult is removed.
In your son's case, if there is pressure by some bone deformity, the removal of this could possibly bring back
function. Note I said *possibly,* not *probably.*

In the meanwhile, you should do all the things which
are conducive to good health of nervous tissue. He needs

*See Product Information.

all the basic vitamins and minerals. In addition, he needs lots of Vitamins C, E, A, B, F. Actually this is really all of the vitamins. Minerals include phosphorus as found in lecithin, magnesium, calcium, as well as all the trace elements. All these are necessary, and enzymes, too. Also, RNA or ribonucleic acid. Large doses of RNA are very useful in correcting nerve damage problems which are thought to be incurable; but it must be taken in large doses over a long period of time.

I've heard that quadriplegics who have nil prognosis have benefited when the extremities were painted daily with DMSO (dimethyl sulfoxide), the persecuted drug. It is denied to humans even though thousands and thousands of case records are available testifying to its beneficial powers. Results of therapy come slowly with DMSO, they say.

Tic Douloureux

Q. *I have suffered from tic douloureux for the past year, and have found nothing to alleviate the pain. A doctor suggested cutting the facial nerve, but I am against that form of torture. Do you have any suggestions for a cure?*—Mrs. L.E.McC., Spokane, Wash.

A. Tic douloureux, or trifacial neuralgia, is a condition in which the trigeminal cranial nerve (fifth cranial nerve) is registering pain for no apparent reason. The pain is usually associated with only one of the three branches of the trigeminal nerve. It is usually persistent in that location, but does spread sometimes to the other branches. The pain is so severe that the patient is willing to undergo drastic treatment for relief.

Treatment usually consists of novocaine or local anesthetic injections at the site of the branch which is causing the trouble. In more severe cases where the local anesthetic does not work for a long enough period of time, absolute alcohol may be injected. This kills the nerve fibers involved for a period of six months or more, as a rule. Gradually the nerve axions regrow into the nerve root and function recurs.

Sometimes the new fibers, or axions, do not get involved

in the neuritic picture again, and the case is cured. Sometimes the new fibers carry on where the old fibers left off. In this case, further injections can be done as needed. The ultimate treatment is a severing of the nerve as suggested by your doctor. This requires the opening of the skull to perform the severance. Patients have to be in severe pain to undergo this type of treatment. Many of them do so gladly for relief.

In all these situations, the fibers of the fifth nerve are temporarily or almost permanently destroyed. This means that functions carried on by the nerve are discontinued. The fifth nerve functions in a sensory capacity of receiving sensations from the face. The most important areas here are the eye and mouth. For instance, the patient cannot tell whether he has anything in his eye or not. In some cases, a foreign body can be in the eye and can be scratching the cornea in a very damaging manner and the patient may not even be aware of it. Or he can be chewing his cheek and not even know it.

Nutritionally some things can be done successfully, sometimes. There should be a good liver detoxification program. The adrenal cortex should be supported too. In addition, one can give plenty of Vitamin B-2 (riboflavin), along with C. Raw nerve tissue extract* is a must. This is an all-out effort, but it can be very rewarding to some who faithfully try.

Facial Paralysis

Q. *My husband suffers from facial paralysis which his doctor said would go away two years ago, but has not. It has affected his right eye and the left side of his mouth and left ear. He has a constant ringing in his ear that is very nerve-racking. We have gone to ear specialists and they tell him there is nothing to be done.*—Mrs. N.P., Waco, Texas.

A. It sounds as if your husband is suffering from Bell's Palsy. This is a condition where there is a paralysis of the facial or 7th cranial nerve. Such paralysis can be brought on by exposure to a cold draft while riding in a car with

*See Product Information.

the window open, or when the face may be exposed on a cold night. Such a paralysis is supposed to be a transient thing and it clears up in a few weeks even without any treatment. However, in my experience, there is usually a residual effect in the motor function of this nerve. It is weak and the muscles droop as a result. One of the first things to do when this condition strikes is to be sure to protect the eye. This is so because the eye many times cannot close properly. It is then subject to dryness or injury. The next thing to do is to keep the facial muscles from drooping too much. This can be done by "splinting" with adhesive tape. Face muscle-strengthening exercise may also help.

Systemically, the approach is to strengthen nerve function. Anything that can be done to improve the nerve function should be used. Vitamin B complex is very valuable, especially B-6. Vitamin E in the form of wheat germ oil could be of great value. Mineral balancing in the tissues should be attempted immediately. Raw nerve tissue extract* should be used abundantly and immediately. Iodine is an antibiotic of sorts in the body so should be used just in case there is a virus present. Iodine in the form of kelp is helpful. Naturally, a complete metabolic checkup is essential.

Nerve Damage

Q. *I've been through surgery twice and also had a vein transplant from my leg to my arm and hand because I had an accident several months ago and cut the leaders in my hand and wrist. They said I was well so I went back to college. Now I find I'm losing strength in my hand and I am going in and out of the hospital for therapy and also learning how to write with my left hand. I am just about going out of my mind with numbness setting in on my right hand. I am 22 years old, and I can't compete in any sport. If there is anything you can tell me to help get strength back in my right hand I'd appreciate it. I can work my fingers a little but can't grip anything. I'll try anything.*—Miss R.W., Cincinnati, Ohio.

*See Product Information.

A. From your statements, I tend to think that you have damaged some of the nerves in the hand. This is causing the numbness. As a second possibility, you may be having some scar tissue forming which is gradually cutting off the circulation as well as causing pressure on the nerves so that they are not functioning properly. In the first place, the nerve tissue will tend to recover and rebuild the axion so that the normal function is reestablished. In the second place, the scar tissue formation can be caused to stop or even recede by the use of Vitamin E. I suspect that large dosages of E will be necessary over a long period of time to accomplish this desired result. Vitamin B-6 (in addition to a full B-complex food such as brewer's yeast) also helps numbness of this type. Brewer's yeast can be added to liquids and consumed once or more daily.

Daily application of the persecuted drug, DMSO, could cause improvement. It is available for horses at your local veterinarian.

Loss of Taste

Q. *For some time I have had a loss of taste. Recently I read an article which said zinc was good for this condition. What is your opinion?*—B. M., Placentia, Ca.

A. To me, loss of taste means that there is some sort of malfunction of the nervous system and, so, I would approach your problem with much effort to enhance nerve function. All the nutrients which are especially involved in nerve function could be used to the maximum. First, a raw nerve tissue extract* to help supply cell regeneration. Next, all the B vitamins are very closely associated with nerve function. Then C to enhance soft tissue action. Nerve tissue is about 20 percent phospholipid in structure so lecithin should be of value. Be sure to compensate for lecithin with adequate calcium since too much lecithin can cause severe calcium deficiency. Zinc may be useful, too.

*See Product Information.

Loss of Taste and Smell

Q. *Last December I lost my taste and smell. It seems incredible, as I live the health way, eating unsprayed foods—and using supplements. Could you please offer a solution to this problem?*—Mrs. C.L.H., Linesville, Pennsylvania.

A. Just living the health way does not exempt you from possible illnesses. One has to look to the nerve function involved in the areas stated. Nerve integrity depends upon a properly balanced nutritional intake as well as adequate B complex, lecithin, calcium, et al. In your situation, I would suggest the possibility of a small stroke in the brain centers involved with these functions. This could be in the form of a little localized hemorrhage or a blood clot there. I can think of no local type of condition that could cause this problem so one must go to the central area to account for all the symptoms involved. Thus the idea of a cerebral lesion.

Myelitis

Q. *My daughter recently became ill with myelitis. Presumably this affects the spinal cord and thus all the muscles, as I understand. The sensation of swelling she experiences is painful, particularly in the back area. Sometimes it's difficult for her to stand on her feet when getting out of bed—or even to open and close her hand. Do you have any suggestions?*—F. H., Anaheim, Ca.

A. Myelitis simply means a type of inflammation of the spinal cord like poliomyelitis or anterolateral myelitis, etc. It is primarily a destruction of the myelin sheath by inflammation. The symptom picture depends upon the location of the lesion and the nerves involved. It could be a paralysis, a sensory problem like excessive pain, etc.

According to the nutritional concept, it is necessary to supply the patient with an abundance of the various nutrients favorable to nerve tissue metabolism. Vitamin B complex is a primary need; so is magnesium chloride which some claim to be a specific for polio. All the minerals including the trace minerals, all vitamins and a generous supply of enzymes are necessary and vital for the myelitic patient. It represents a total program now and forever.

A 10:1 wheat germ oil preparation which supposedly contains basic elements necessary to heal nerve degenerative states is now on the market. It contains the neuromuscular factor. The dosage is large and the treatment period is long, therefore quite expensive. However, how does one measure expense at a time like this? Magnesium chloride may help.

Numbness in Toes

Q. *Recently my husband went to the doctor because his second toe on both feet were ever so slightly numb. He checked his cholesterol, said it was high (270) and also said he was a little anemic. He suggested high dosages of natural vitamins. He also recommended a high protein-low fat diet. I was wondering whether the high dosages of Vitamin E and C are not a little too much. Also, I just read that you do not approve of dolomite for calcium. I gather you do approve of bone meal.*—Mrs. D. K., Bronx, New York.

A. It could be a deterioration of a nerve tissue as a result of lack of Vitamin B-12 and folic acid, like in pernicious anemia. It also could be due to a lack of Vitamin B-6 since B-6 affects the nerve endings in fingers and toes.

Vitamin E, needed for circulation, is also a possibility. Every person has his own dosage or need of Vitamin E. It seems to me that a starting dosage of 300 units working upward gradually until symptoms cease, is the proper approach.

Vitamin C may help, too. According to studies made by the orthomolecular group, it is felt that 5,000 mg per day is the amount needed just for average living, 15,000 mg if the stress is not too great but up to 100,000 mg if there is major stress.

No, I do not approve of dolomite of the White Cliffs of Dover. The cliffs certainly are natural, but not organic. I would use raw bone meal tablets.* Dosage depends upon how much is in the tablets and how much the patient needs.

Burning Feet

Q. *Would you please tell me what causes my feet to burn at night? This does not occur every night, but when it does, I am unable to sleep. I have been told it is caused by an allergy, and also that it is due to kidney trouble, but the doctor says my kidneys are O.K. I am 79 years old.—* A.L.B., Petersburg, Tex.

A. It would seem that a simple symptom like burning feet would be easy to explain. On the contrary, it is rather complex. The cause could be circulatory, hormonal or neural. For example, there could be significant hardening of the arteries so that the circulation is reduced and the consumption of oxygen is much below the normal level. There could be poor venous drainage of the limbs, so that the tissues become congested. There could be a shortage of Vitamin E. This vitamin not only improves the delivery of oxygen to the area, but also improves the utilization of the oxygen after it gets there. The same is true of Vitamin B-15.

Among the nervous problems would be the deficiency of calcium or vitamins niacinamide and pyridoxine (Vitamin B-6). Also, do not forget the menopausal syndrome. This could show itself in just such a manner. Even an allergic condition could be the basic cause here.

What is needed in such a condition is to have a complete metabolic examination followed by a knowledgeable nutritional therapeutic program.

It has finally dawned on me that hot feet at night is a symptom of thyroid malfunction. This symptom should subside with adequate iodine therapy—say 1 drop per day of half water and half tincture of iodine. This supplies about 1.0 mg iodine per day. It takes several months for this therapy to become effective.

*See Product Information.

Motion Sickness

Q. *I am 75 years of age and have been troubled with motion sickness all my life when I travel as a passenger. I can drive myself all day without the least trouble. Is there anything I can do to overcome this trouble? I am getting to the age when travelling in congested areas and at high speed is tiring.*—J.S.B., Carlisle, Pa.

A. Motion sickness is probably due to lack of B complex vitamins in the nerve tissue. The nutritional approach would be to make sure that there is an adequate intake of the complex, that there is adequate digestion of the substances, that there is proper absorption, metabolism and excretion of these various substances. Vitamin B-6, in addition to the entire B complex, has been helpful to some.

Another possible cause of motion sickness might be the shortage of calcium in the nerve cells. Maybe other trace mineral imbalances could cause the same sort of symptom complex reaction, too. So seriously consider Vitamin B complex, Vitamin B-6, calcium and other trace minerals in connection with your problem.

37. Nose

Nosebleeds

Q. *I have been diagnosed as having telangiectasis, which in my case is a family problem—four or five of us of a large family have this disorder. I have had electrocoagulation many times from a specialist; another specialist recommended only vaseline. Still I have daily nosebleeds. Four or five years ago a doctor diagnosed rheumatoid arthritis and after several years of medicine I decided to drop all drugs and treat myself with corrected diet and vitamin supplements. I no longer have arthritis with my improved regimen, but I have not found the cure-all for nosebleeds. Lately, they are becoming worse, increasing from several a day to sometimes off and on all day—interfering with my job and resulting in constantly stuffed and coagulated nasal passages. Do you have any suggestions?*—A.M.W., Independence, Mo.

A. I think your clue is the association of nosebleeds with rheumatoid arthritis. The two could have a common cause. My first bet is a deficiency of the Vitamin C complex (bioflavonoids). This is not ascorbic acid but the whole natural Vitamin C complex. I know you tried this, but I am a firm believer in brand names since all products, even with the same labels, are not the same. Maybe the product you used is good if combined with large amounts of the natural complex. I think it would be worth another try. B complex also helps.

Another item which could give you help is Vitamin E. Again the natural form is preferable. Natural Vitamin E is in wheat germ oil. Assuming you have good liver function, you could take up to a tablespoonful four times daily for a while then cut it down when the load of oil becomes too much.

318

Nosebleeds can also be caused by food allergies, or allergies from air and household products, pillows etc. High blood pressure is another cause.

Nasal Polyps

Q. *During the past four years, I have had nasal polyps removed five times. The doctor has diagnosed the problem as hyperplastic sinusitis—nasal polyposis.*

I will be very grateful if you will please advise me whether something can be done nutritionally, plus vitamins and minerals, to prevent the regrowth of the polyps.— H.Z., Berwyn, Ill.

A. Nasal polyposis of this duration is a gigantic problem. All possible types of solutions concerning this malady must be applied with vigor in order to get the desired results.

First, the diet must be completely devoid of anything that can be aggravating to the nasal mucosa. This usually means the absence of all highly processed carbohydrates, canned foods, foods containing chemical preservatives, as well as all known allergens.

Next, make sure that there is an abundant intake of good, natural Vitamin C. Vitamin A intake must be adequate, also.

The liver must be functioning in good order. This means that the patient should go through a complete and extensive liver detoxification program. The use of natural antihistamines can be considered. My favorite is the liver hormone, yakriton.*

Any substance that will help to improve oxygen saturation of the blood and tissues is of great value here. These items include, among others, balanced intakes of Vitamins E and B complex. Sometimes the nucleic tissue extracts, primarily the mucous membrane tissue extract from the respiratory tract, do a good job in rebuilding tissue. This substance is available from companies in the United States and is listed as raw lung tissue extract.*

Every avenue of possible benefit should be explored in this particular problem.

Nasal polyps respond well to other antiallergic modali-

*See Product Information.

ties. A simple one, five drops of castor oil taken in juice by mouth in water upon arising, tends to cut down the histaminic reaction. Heparin has an antihistaminic reaction too. I use a long-acting, water-soluble form, 500 units by hypo twice weekly. This causes a gradual subsiding of the polyps.

As a last resort, polyps may be removed surgically. This is a simple office procedure for the most part. Of course this does not solve the cause, but does eliminate the results for a while, at least.

Polyps

Q. *Could you please tell me what causes polyps? Does it come from a vitamin deficiency?*—S.P., Tampa, Fla.

A. Nasal polyps are caused by the mucous membranes of the nose becoming waterlogged and then drooping down into the passage. In this instance the polyp is simply normal tissue which has become supersaturated with water. It is an allergic reaction.

The chances are that your daughter is allergic to milk, chocolate and/or wheat. Another factor may be a deficiency of calcium and Vitamin D. Extensive work in this area has been done by Dr. Carl Reich, M.D., of Calgary, Canada. He has done wonderful work with severe respiratory allergic cases with the use of Vitamin D and calcium. Vitamins A, C, bioflavonoids as well as D and calcium are important. In fact, the total intake must be in harmony, which means that *all* nutrients are needed.

Atrophic Rhinitis

Q. *Is atrophic rhinitis due to a nutritional vitamin or mineral deficiency? If so, what is lacking?*—H.Z., Berwyn, Ill.

A. Atrophic rhinitis is a condition where the mucous membrane of the nasal passages has undergone atrophy. (Atrophy is a condition where the tissue has begun to deteriorate or to become less virile.) It is comparable to the atrophy of muscles when a cast is applied to the arms for a period of time and the muscles become weak and smaller in size. When the mucous membrane of the nose begins to atrophy, it becomes thinner and less active in its secretory action. Each individual cell shrinks up a bit or dries out a little.

I would say very definitely that this condition is associated with nutritional deficiencies. The main problem is to determine just what is out of order. As to other types of deficiencies, what is *your* particular problem is not necessarily the problem of the next patient. This is why it is necessary to go through a complete analysis in each case. Some deficiencies are a little more likely to cause certain problems, but this is by no means a rule of thumb.

Regarding the rhinitis, it is safe to say that the need for Vitamin A is very basic, as is the need for the bioflavonoid group. All the minerals are essential, especially potassium, calcium and sodium. The aim is to get a proper balance to the tissues. Also, one cannot ignore the protein balance. Even if there are enough minerals and vitamins, if protein is not present, then proper healing cannot take place.

Even if all items are present, it still takes the metabolism of the tissue to utilize them, so if the condition has been present for a long period, it takes much more effort and much more time to correct the imbalance.

38. Respiratory Problems

Emphysema

Q. *When I had a recent examination, the doctor told me I had pulmonary emphysema and that there was nothing that could be done about it. Will you please advise if there is anything that I can do that would help the condition? I never did smoke, but many years ago I worked in a chemical plant where I had to breathe fumes that hurt me a lot at the time. I am 76 years of age.*—M.O.L., Bakersfield, Calif.

A. Emphysema is a condition in the lungs where the small air sacs, or alveoli, have ruptured into one another so that there are fewer, but larger air sacs than originally. This results in a lessening of the tissue surface contact with respired air. Thus, there is a difficulty in bringing oxygen into the body and in removing waste products through the lungs. In your case, the causative factor of great importance is, no doubt, the heavy exposure to chemicals.

Treatment is not so hopeless as the allopathic doctors are led to believe. Naturally, there can be no regeneration of tissue once it has been destroyed, as in the rupturing of the air sacs. However, there is almost always an associated infection in the lungs. The situation can be eased somewhat by building up the ability of the body to manufacture better antibodies. This can be accomplished by using a nucleic acid preparation of raw thymus tissue*. The lung tissue can also be strengthened to a certain degree by consumption of raw lung nucleic acid preparations.*

Vitamin C is the kingpin to the defensive mechanisms, so it should be taken in adequate, or greater, dosages. Vitamin E will improve the utilization ratio of the available oxygen. So will Vitamin B-15. Ammonium chloride will

*See Product Information.

help to allay the effects of the respiratory alkalosis which invariably develops in such a condition.*

These are some of the approaches which should be combined with a nutritional program to build up the entire body.

See also breathing suggestions under "Hyperventilation."

Bronchial Asthma

Q. *Our grandmother, who is not quite 66 years old, is suffering very much lately from bronchial asthma. She also has an enlarged heart. She sees her doctor regularly and takes pills every day, which give her some relief. She would be thankful for any advice you could give her concerning her diet.*—Mrs. R.K., Denver, Colo.

A. This is a very unfortunate situation. An already overworked heart must do extra duty in face of the asthmatic lungs—an almost unbearable situation. The first step would be a thorough metabolic evaluation of the patient as a whole. For instance, if she were checked in 500 routine checkpoints and properly evaluated, the doctor would know more about her than if he evaluated only 100 checkpoints. This is the ultimate value of the survey type of health evaluation. Often small variations from normal mean the real difference between success and failure. Many times doctors treat successfully the main problem, but fail in the minor ones.

It is my guess that this woman suffers from liver failure to a significant degree. She also may have a failure of the adrenal cortex glands, in addition to the obvious heart and lung failures. There is probably kidney damage, too. So you see that there must be a total approach to your grandmother's case.

First, I would put her on a very restricted diet, like a grape diet or carrot juice diet or grapefruit and celery. One or two foods which do not cause her trouble should be selected. These would be eaten eight times daily for a period of two, three or four weeks. Of course, she should be under close supervision and should have adequate food

*See Product Information.

supplements to ensure adequate nutritional intake. These supplements should include the various raw tissue extracts which are indicated in her case as determined by her history and checkup.

After control has been obtained, her diet could be expanded slowly to be sure not to overload the functions of the system. As she demonstrates her capability, her diet can gradually enlarge, but if and when symptoms develop, an immediate withdrawal is in order concerning the dietary program. Incidentally, many times this dietary can ultimately contain items which were thought to be forbidden for life, since the tissues are now rebuilt functionally. There is much hope for a patient such as the one mentioned in this question, if the program is handled properly.

Susceptibility to Colds, Etc.

Q. *For most of my 28 years, I have had colds, bronchitis, flu and, last year, pneumonia. Can you advise me?*—Miss G., Washington, D.C.

A. Naturally, a complete metabolic analysis is in order to ascertain the details of your nutritional needs. There is always something that the individual needs to correct in such a situation.

In addition, it is quite possible that you have an organism or group of organisms which you have harbored in your system for a long time. Your system does not have the strength to force out the infection. Yet the organism is not virulent enough to cause a steady illness. Antibiotics are not sufficiently strong to completely eradicate the infection, but only strong enough to cause the acuteness of the infection to partially subside. In such a case, it could be very wise to get a culture of the offending organisms and to have autogenous vaccines made. These vaccines can then be taken by mouth over a long period of time, starting with a minute dosage and gradually increasing it until the body is able to cope with the infection.

The technique is similar to animal methods. They lick the wounds and take the offending germs into their systems so their bodies can be stimulated to generate the appropriate antibiotics to eradicate the infection. This treatment can take as long as five years, but is worth the effort since there appears to be no other way to cleanse the body of such offenders.

Influenza Epidemic

Q. *My husband recently contracted the flu and developed pneumonia. He responded dramatically to the penicillin the doctor gave him. Is there any damage to the lungs because he has had pneumonia? While he was sick, he would eat nothing but eggnogs with raw honey, lecithin granules and yeast with milk.*—W.L., Coeur d'Alene, Idaho.

A. To the best of my knowledge, it would appear that he does not have any permanent damage to his lungs, although it is true that the tissues have been insulted.

The diet you gave him while he was sick is not good. He should have been on clear juices only. This may be why he developed the penumonia. The body should be relieved of the task of digesting heavy foods while it is sick and trying to eliminate the accumulated toxins.

Clear fluids will sustain the patient while he is sick. If extra feeding is needed, and it is a good idea anyway, feed the body through the skin. Simply rub apple cider vinegar into the skin at frequent intervals. He can also be fed through the rectum. The use of an enema containing two tablespoonfuls each of honey and lemon juice can readily aid in the support of the body while it is sick. I have even used large dosages of 1:1000 intravenous injections of hydrochloric acid for the treatment of serious infections when the patient is allergic to penicillin or other antibiotics. Maybe even 20cc of this 1:1000 mixture can be given slowly at one time. It has the power of penicillin on occasion.

Hyperventilation

Q. *I wonder if you could tell me how to alleviate a condition diagnosed as hyperventilation.*—E.B., Brooklyn, New York.

A. Hyperventilation is a problem brought on by heart or lung conditions, in which the patient breathes rapidly with the chest held in extension. This causes a very rapid excretion of carbon dioxide from the lungs, which in turn causes respiratory alkalosis. Alkalosis causes more hyperventilation. The circle is complete and can actually result in such serious problems as a heart attack.

The first step is to make the patient exhale completely. This may require several breaths and continued monitoring for a while. He can be helped by placing a hand firmly on the chest pressing downward with each expiration. As the chest is held in the deflated position, the patient is encouraged to breathe with the abdomen. Slow, deep breathing is the goal.

After some control is restored it would be wise to have a complete metabolic examination especially of the heart including the electrocardiogram, phonocardiogram and plethysmograph.

Fibrosis of the Lungs

Q. *I have a disease the doctors tell me is terminal. They do not know when. It is a lung disease. A fibrosis of some sort—breathing is very difficult. It may be foolish at this stage of the game to be looking for help as medicine says they have no cure as they don't know the cause.*—M.G., La Mesa, California.

A. The condition you are trying to explain is a fibrosis of the lungs where the normal lung tissue is being replaced by the fibrous tissue which has no pulmonary function. It simply fills in the gaps and does not allow the normal tissue to function properly. As this progresses, your ability to breathe decreases.

There is nothing known to help you in the orthodox medical field. However, in the nutritional approach, there may be some ray of hope. I have no idea as to how much, but do know that at least you can be relieved of some of your suffering. My first suggestion would be to administer large dosages of Vitamin C. Most of this should be given intravenously since the G.I. tract would not be capable of tolerating from 10 to 30 grams of Vitamin C daily.

Naturally, this dosage of Vitamin C must be accompanied by appropriate doses of calcium. Even if this sort of dosage did not help with the primary condition, it, at least, would make life more bearable by relieving pain and other distress. My second suggestion would be to administer raw pulmonary tissue extract. This is the extract of lung tissue.* This contains the RNA and DNA of the lung and tends to help the lung tissue to normalize. Naturally, all the basic vitamins and minerals are indicated in this therapy, too. The administration of raw thymus tissue extract would increase ability to produce resistance. . . . So would thymus tissue in the sense that the blood count (lymphocytes) could be increased.

I would also give the preparation known as SPL or Staphage Lysate. I would administer this in 0.1cc intradermal doses on a tri-weekly basis. It could be that subcutaneous doses of 0.5cc would be more in conformity to the urgency of the situation.

Another injection of great potential value is the one I call D&L. This is made by mixing 1cc of crude liver extract with 3½cc 2% novocaine into 100cc pure distilled water. The dosage is 1cc per 25 pounds of body weight given intramuscularly using a 23g needle in sites not to exceed 2½cc each. This injection also given three times weekly should contribute to healing of the lesion.

At least these are some of the starters for a so-called incurable condition which could possibly become curable.

*See Product Information.

39. Sinus

Sinusitis

Q. *For 25 years I have had what the doctors call sinusitis, although the intense pain is in my temple. It beats like a hammer at times and seems to go down in my ear tube. However, my nose does stop up. I take a lot of drugs such as aspirin, Empirin, B.C.'s, etc., hoping the pain will stop. This, in turn, gives me butterflies in my stomach and I am in a miserable fix. The attacks last two or three days at a time. Can you tell me what to do?*

I have been taking yeast; 50,000 units of Vitamin A; 4000 units of Vitamin D; 300 or 400 units of Vitamin E; one B-complex tablet; 8 dolomite tablets; and 8 calcium tablets per day. I take vinegar and honey twice a day. I have had no cooked food except millet for 12 years. (I am 55). I don't use white salt, but use Vegetal. I do not use white sugar, white flour or cereals and eat very little bread of any kind. What can I do? I am desperate.— J.E.L., Atlanta, Ga.

A. You need a complete liver detoxification program. You also, more than likely, suffer from hypoglycemia and should avail yourself of proper management of this condition. I would suggest that you go on a mono or duo diet for a couple of weeks. By this, I mean eat only one or two foods during this period. I would pick a food like grapes, watermelon, carrot juice, grapefruit and celery or some such combination which fits your economy and can be readily obtained in the fresh state, preferably "organically" grown.

Supplements should be used wisely. Vitamins C, A, bioflavonoids, calcium are needed; and, of course, the whole balanced program is important. Some recent work seems to indicate that RNA is of great value in restoring tissue to normal levels. Raw lung (and respiratory tract tissue) extracts are of great value, too.*

Contrary to the strict nutritional approach, I do feel that there is a definite place for nose drops or sprays. Complications arise when there is inadequate drainage of the sinuses. Sprays insure adequate drainage, even though there is a price to pay for their use. Nasal sprays of a solution of aqueous chlorophyll can be used alternately (two days on and one day off) with a dilute solution of apple cider vinegar solution. The chlorophyll solution can be made by dissolving the contents of one capsule of aqueous chlorophyll in two ounces of distilled water. The vinegar solution consists of one teaspoonful of apple cider vinegar in two ounces of distilled water.

Five drops of castor oil in water first thing in the morning can be very beneficial. So also heparin shots as described elsewhere in this book.

The combination of all these measures seems to be of value in the treatment of this condition.

Sinus Headaches

Q. *I would like to know about sinus headaches. Do you know of any natural ways to find relief?*—J.W., Kansas City, Mo.

A. You could try niacin, because I believe it could be of value. You could also try Vitamin C and pantothenic acid. In large doses these can and do aid in alleviating allergic and infectious conditions in the nasal passages including the sinuses. In extreme cases, I would give up to 1,000 mg hourly of C and maybe 1,000 mg of pantothenic acid four to six times daily. After control is obtained, the dosages can be reduced.

Post Nasal Drip

Q. *Will you please help me nutritionally with a bronchial problem, allergy, post nasal drip and hay fever. I've had it for years and nothing has helped at all.*—Mrs. H.C.S., Houston, Texas.

*See Product Information.

A. Basically, you need to have much more acid in your system, mainly hydrochloric acid, although there are other forms which would be satisfactory. You could also take organic vinegar from apples or grapes as an adjunct to your intake of food. The second major item needed is calcium. This is needed in the acid based form. Over a period of time, this will correct the deficiency in your system. As an adjunct to this one could take a magnesium orotate.*

Halitosis and Sinus

Q. *I'm writing about a chronic problem that has plagued me for as long as I can remember. I have bad breath morning, noon and night. I chew gum, suck mints and use mouth washes constantly. Nothing helps. My tongue is usually coated. I also have a post nasal drip which nothing cures. Sinus condition has been my constant companion. I take 50,000 units A, B complex, C—all day—E, 600 units, a calcium and mineral tablet. I just don't know what else to do.*—Mrs. A.K., Flint, Michigan.

A. Halitosis usually comes from some sort of local condition such as bad gums, chronic throat infection, chronic sinusitis, etc. It also comes from such lung diseases as pneumonia, tuberculosis, abscesses of lung and all sorts of conditions. It also comes from intestinal tract conditions such as ulcers, gastritis, inflamed intestinal tract, gallbladder disease, diverticulitis and all sorts of other conditions of the gastrointestinal diseases. Since you mention the sinus condition, this is probably your answer. Sinusitis which has been present for a great number of years is more difficult than that which has been present for a shorter period.

One of the most basic answers to chronic sinusitis is to establish drainage of the sinus. Mechanically this can be done by finger manipulation of the nasopharynx, probing upward toward the Eustachian tube. Finger manipulation of the nasal passages helps a lot. Using a local anesthetic on the gloved finger, the nose may be probed and opened

*See Product Information.

gently. A finger cot used as a balloon can be suddenly inflated in the nasal passage and held in the inflated position for a moment will do wonders to open the passages. This type of treatment should be used daily for the best results.

40. Skin

Scleroderma

Q. *By biopsy a spot about two by four inches on the right side of my back was diagnosed as morphea type scleroderma three years ago. I use or have used various creams or oil on it to help it from being so dry—including comfrey, Vitamin E oil, aloe vera gel, and also others. I take natural food supplements like whole B but I am wondering whether I should take extra amounts of certain others? Also what can you tell me about this disease?—* W.J.H., Scotts Valley, Ca.

A. Scleroderma is a systemic disease which may involve the connective tissue of the body, including the skin, heart, esophagus, kidney and lung. The skin may be thickened, hard, rigid and pigmented patches may occur. There is no known cause for this condition and there is supposedly no cure known.

Nutritionally speaking, there are a few things that can be done. General support measures for overall health are needed. This includes the intake of the basic vitamins and minerals. Next, it is necessary to have the information from a complete metabolic examination so that each major system of the body is evaluated and support measures can be taken to the extent as indicated. This means that the nerves are supported for optimal function; the cardiovascular system, the digestive system and all others are supported likewise.

The skin is particularly important in this condition so it needs the greatest support. By support, I mean that the need of the particular tissue involved is particularly supported. The need of skin is not the same as heart or brain, etc. The variety of nutrients of each cell and tissue are the same but the balance is different for each. Skin is particularly "hungry" for Vitamin B complex, Vitamins A and

D, minerals like zinc and manganese and Vitamin C. Since the condition involves hardening of the tissues, one suspects that calcium is a prominent figure among the causative factors. The use of magnesium is especially important in the metabolism of calcium.

Scleroderma

Q. *I am in need of information about scleroderma. The most information I have been able to find is in Adelle Davis' book* Let's Get Well. *If there is any more, I need to learn all I can.*—Mrs. H. P., Bellevue, Michigan.

A. It may seem very strange to many people and quite out of context to the orthodox way of thinking but there is no set answer to any condition. What is important is that every person is different. There are no two people alike in the whole world. Just like fingerprints, the whole individual body is unique. Even the biochemical and metabolic manner of action is different. In my office we try to determine your individualities. Then we try to support the normal actions, and to make abnormal ones more normal. When this is accomplished, the living organism, known as the body, can make the corrections itself. No drug or vitamin has ever cured anything. It is the body which cures itself, but it must be supplied with the necessary raw materials (vitamins, minerals, etc.) with which to make the normalizing corrections.

So, scleroderma is no different from other conditions ... treatment depends upon individuality of patients.

A relatively new treatment for the hardening diseases is the use of EDTA. This is a complicated process which should only be administered by those particularly trained in the technique. It consists of a series of intravenous injections of EDTA, usually about 20 in number. This material chelates the available ionic calcium from the blood stream and excretes it through the kidneys. With this void of calcium in the blood stream, some of the calcium from the hardened tissues becomes ionic and passes into the blood where it can be removed by chelation in each successive treatment. There are many possible complications and unknowns about this form of treatment so it must be handled by a doctor with great caution. I do believe that chelation therapy would be a benefit in this condition.

Psoriasis

Q. *We are hopeful you can provide information about treatment of psoriasis for our 5-year-old grandson. He incidentally has a twin brother who is not affected. The child is in excellent health otherwise, emotionally stable, and he has a good home environment. Unfortunately, his diet is typically American—consisting of dry breakfast cereals, sweets, condiments and soft drinks, though, of course, we disapprove. The child, however, seems to enjoy fresh fruits and vegetables when offered or available. I have been sending a Vitamin E ointment which is applied locally to scalp and legs. This seems to help somewhat, but exacerbations are still common. Could you give any suggestions or comments regarding a diet or supplement program he might follow?—H.S.*

A. You give the nature of the condition, in fact, diagnosed for us and then go on to give the cause and treatment. One can wonder why the other twin is not affected. I cannot give the answer. There must be some difference in hereditary traits so that the one reacts more unfavorably to the noxious stimuli of the usual American diet while the other is not so sensitive. People are this way: some are very sensitive to a given situation while others are hardly sensitive at all.

This child needs all the available resources of the nutritional approach. He needs a total nutritional rehabilitation and rebuilding program. Lecithin has been used in many cases for relief of psoriasis. Zinc may be a specific type of treatment.

Psoriasis

Q. *What health food or vitamin can I take to help rid my skin of psoriasis? I am 45 and have had psoriasis off and on since I was 16.*

I have tried granular lecithin, but found out my cholesterol count was normal, so discontinued it. Am now trying Vitamin C—1000 milligrams a day. I think it helps. If nothing else, I don't catch colds.—Mrs. J.B., Los Angeles, Calif.

A. Psoriasis is in reality a systemic disease, and no matter what and how much of something you put on the skin, you will not solve the problem. The first essential is for you to have a complete metabolic survey. This will give definite leads as to what your special needs are. The cause of psoriasis in your case may be quite different than the causative factors in the next case. Each case is individual unto himself.

However, one of the factors which usually is contributory to such a situation is the lack of zinc. You must be careful about zinc, even as you are careful about which vitamins you take. Not all vitamins are the same, even if they are all sold in the health food stores.

Minerals, to do the best job, must be organic. This means that they must be combined with certain organic compounds such as proteins, aminoacids, etc. They are not inorganic, or combined with certain elements like chloride, nitrate, sulfate, etc.

Unfortunately, you, as a buyer, cannot read the labels and determine which product is the one you want. The labeling laws are weighted in favor of the manufacturer who wishes to get away with as much as possible and still make you believe he is saying the product contains the factors you are looking for.

Melasma

Q. *I have a skin condition called melasma which first appeared five and a half years after continuous use of the birth control pill. Six months after it first appeared I discontinued using the Pill. Nevertheless, it has been getting worse each of the three summers since. Do you have any comments or suggestions to offer?*—J.M., Worcester, Mass.

A. I am not sure that the Pill caused your condition, but the coincidence is remarkable. I first think in terms of total nutrition. Cells need all vitamins, minerals and enzymes at each meal to make the metabolic machinery go. If you are in need of Vitamin B complex, and I believe you are, you should first think of the basic B complex as found in yeast and liver, for instance. Also, add enough B-6 to the program. PABA is one more member of the B complex you should investigate.

Another grave oversight in your program is lack of B-12. Folic acid and B-12 are needed together when used therapeutically. Lack of B-12 could allow neurological damage to progress unchecked in cases of pernicious anemia.

Keloid Scars

Q. *Keloid scars (hypertrophy) are described as "benign tumors." Is there ever danger of malignancy? What causes them? Why would one-half of an incision heal normally and the other half become a keloid scar? Surgeons advise excision, X ray, and/or cortisone injections into the scar tissue as the only methods of removal. But there is a possibility of recurrence. Is there any way to avoid keloid scars?*—Mrs. C.B.S., Hillcrest Heights, Maryland.

A. There are two major types of tumors: benign and malignant. The former is not malignant and does not generally develop into a malignancy. Keloids are scars on the skin which are very large and stick out above the level of the surrounding skin. They are considered disfiguring, but not dangerous in relation to a malignancy possibility. I cannot speculate why you have part of the scar involved and not the other. It would do no good to have them excised, because they will very likely form again. X ray will stop the development and may even reduce it. However, you are taking a chance on the level of X-ray dosage needed which might cause cancer in the surrounding tissues. Cortisone injections are worthless in the long run.

Nutritionally, one should be sure to have enough of the unsaturated fatty acids in the diet as well as applying them locally. (These products are known by the name of Vitamin F.) The function here is to help metabolize fats properly in the body.

Herpes Simplex

Q. *Have you any suggestions for herpes simplex? I get these on different parts of my body. My doctor prescribed antibiotics, but they don't seem to be very effective.*—J.T., Toronto, Ontario, Canada.

A. Herpes simplex is a localized virus infection usually involving the tissues around the mouth or nose. My usual approach is the local application of some sort of substance, such as camphor, to dehydrate the lesion. Systemic approach would include the use of copious amounts of Vitamins C and A. Large dosages of lecithin, taken on a limited-time basis, are sometimes dramatically helpful. For instance, take 4000 milligrams of lecithin every 10 minutes for three doses. These three doses may be repeated in six hours or so. If it is necessary to take more than this, be sure to protect yourself with adequate calcium to balance the phosphorus in the lecithin.

Another approach is to use large doses of iodine. My favorite product contains iodine from sea sponge but one may substitute kelp if he desires. The dosage is to take one or two tablets each hour until nervousness begins to develop. At this time the dosage is drastically reduced but maintained sufficiently to give more antiviral effect from the iodine for as long a period as is necessary.

Shingles

Q. *I am just recovering from an eight-week bout with shingles, about which I can find little information. My book says it is herpes zoster and is bilateral but no specific treatment is mentioned. Why is it bilateral? How do you get it, from air, food, water or skin puncture? Can you have it more than once?*—W. T. B., Georgetown, Kentucky.

A. Herpes zoster is a virus infection closely related to chicken pox. It involves the nerve root in an area usually unilateral (one sided) and not bilateral (two sided) as you suggest. The area of involvement is the distribution area of the nerve root involved. The rash occurs usually where this nerve root comes to the surface of the skin. The skin serviced by this nerve usually is quite sore.

In my estimation the treatment is to eliminate the virus infection by using copious amounts of Vitamin C, much lecithin balanced with calcium, large amounts of the Vitamin B complex ... all these done right now with the greatest urgency. An adjunct to the oral approach would be the injection of Vitamin B-12 along with a denatured proteolytic enzyme. Daily injections of this combination tend to bring the herpes under control soon. Otherwise an untreated case of herpes can go along for many months of suffering.

Shingles

Q. *I have had shingles for months and still suffer from a great deal of pain. Do you have any suggestions?*—Mrs. A.E.S., Los Angeles, Calif.

A. Shingles or herpes zoster is another type of neuritis caused by a virus infection. It is a first cousin to chicken pox. It can become very severe and is certainly painful while active. If left alone, it can be very active for many months. The main treatment is the B complex (vitamins). I use large doses including injections of B-12 and folic acid along with enzymes as found in the product Protamide. Raw brain or nerve tissue is indicated for definitive treatment, too. I would also use SPL (Staphage Lysate) injections. This is a staph-antigen-type preparation which tends to build resistance toward staph infections. I also give injections of my D&L solution. This, as mentioned before, is a mixture of 100cc pure distilled water plus 1cc of crude liver extract and 3½cc of two percent procaine, given at a rate of 1cc per 25 lbs. of body weight in intramuscular sites of not more than 2½cc per site. A 23g needle is used for this.

Lupus Erythematosus

Q. *I am a lupus erythematosus victim who regained good health by using good nutrition, positive thinking, knowing all I could learn about my disease. I began my long trail back to good health by drinking one quart of carrot juice a day for a month; one pint a day for a month; then one cup a day for two years. I also began taking the health supplements and still do. At present, I am in very good health.*—Mrs. B.H., Corpus Christi, Texas.

A. If carrot juice has done so much for you in the past, why do you not continue taking it? It seems a little absurd to me. The skin is very much affected by the amount of Vitamin A you get into the body. I would strongly suggest that you take abundant amounts of this vitamin. Of course, the associated intake of Vitamin D is indicated. Cod liver oil is a very good source of this material.

Ruptured Capillaries

Q. *Lately, I have been noticing small, red broken veins (or capillaries) on my cheeks and around my nose. I am quite concerned about these and would like to prevent them from getting any worse.*—Mrs. R.C.

A. These small broken veins are a sign of weakness of the capillary structure. This can be prevented or corrected usually by the use of bioflavonoids in large doses. They are also a sign of liver complications which would respond to a liver detoxification program. In order to find the specific nature of the treatment to be used, a complete metabolic evaluation must be available. The liver has about 300 different functions within the body, some of which can be perfectly normal, while others may be extremely deficient.

What you need is a strong liver detoxification program and a generous intake of the bioflavonoids.

Scar Tissue

Q. *Would the taking of Vitamin E, plus its application to scar tissue following circumcision have any effect in removing it?*—F.L.F., Cincinnati, Ohio.

A. This is an unfortunate place for scar tissue to develop. However, these tissues are no different than any other tissues. The local application of a good mixed tocopherol Vitamin E preparation should soften up the scar tissue and allow for normal healing. It would also help to have an abundant intake of this vitamin by mouth.

Red Blotches

Q. *I am 44 years old, in good health, take all natural vitamins and try to eat a wholesome diet. However, 17 years ago I noticed this blotchy condition on my legs. Red blotches which disappear when I rub the skin or elevate my legs. Sometimes they just disappear by themselves without any apparent reason. Could you give me any suggestions to follow for this situation?*—M., Brooklyn, New York.

A. Exactly where and what your circulatory condition is now is difficult to determine. However, you should be helped greatly by increased intake of the antioxidant vitamins. They are the oil soluble Vitamin E and the water soluble Vitamin C. Naturally, you need a strong basic vitamin intake, but these two should be supplemented in large dosages. If your blood pressure is high you should be a little cautious about the sudden high dosage of Vitamin E. Begin it at lower doses and increase gradually weekly.

Acne

Q. *I have a very severe acne problem which I've had for many years. I'm now 26 and it's still going strong. I've gone to many dermatologists, have been on antibiotics for several years, have had X-ray treatments and been on the Pill—*

all to no avail. I have been watching my diet constantly—I rarely eat meat, stick to basically natural foods and do a lot of yoga—all this hasn't helped. I'm now going to a cosmetologist who cleans and cares for my skin with natural products (cucumber cream, etc.), still my skin breaks out. I'm at the end of my rope. Can you recommend something?—B.M., Huntington, New York.

A. Acne is a plague to teenagers and sometimes into the 20s.

Brewer's yeast taken daily has helped many acne sufferers.

My next approach would be to use methods to eradicate the infection from the body. My first choice here is SPL or Staphage Lysate. This is a vaccine made from the phaged culture of Staph. I would use it intradermally once weekly until resistance is developed. Another injection of value is the one I call D&L. This is simply a mixture of pure distilled water, 100cc with 1cc of crude liver extract and 3½cc of 2 percent procaine. This is administered in intramuscular injections of 1cc per 25 pounds of body weight in sites not to contain more than 2½cc each. This regimen along with the dietary approach could bring your acne under control within a few months.

Fungus Infection

Q. *I am a 50-year-old woman, married, live on a ranch and work in an office at a paper mill (but have no contact with chemicals). For 10 months I have been miserable with a very swollen tongue, generally coated with sores on it and the lining of my mouth. One doctor gave it a name of "erythema multiforme" as I also started getting small red blisters under the skin of my hands that eventually dry up without breaking and then peel. He felt this was related to my mouth trouble and ordered an upper and lower GI that showed nothing. Doctors have put me on fungus medicines, penicillin, cortisone, antihistamines, various mouth washes, Vitamin B complex and Lactinex. Lately I've been on a program of my own, adding anything I've heard or read might be helpful. Nothing I've read exactly describes my case.*

The Lactinex tablets had helped me more than anything, but not permanently, so I felt it was a digestive problem. I am now taking: acidophilus; all vitamins—daily dosage of A (12,500 units), D (1,650 units), E, d-alpha (200 i.u.) all B vitamins (50 mg each), C (at least 1,000 mg), pantothenic acid (300 mg), folic acid (0.1 mg), mineral tablet one with each meal; a protein digestant tablet with each meal that contains five grains of hydrochloric acid; and two tablets at mealtime of natural digestive enzymes for protein, starch and fat. Two weeks ago I started taking one capsule of comfrey-pepsin after meals. I also get an estrogen shot every three weeks for the past five years.

My mouth stays clear of sores for a few weeks then flares up again, but my tongue never has resumed its natural size and stays coated, sometimes worse than others, but not actually discolored or "geographic."

I feel there is some cause that I am not absorbing what I should. I can't take over one teaspoon of brewer's yeast at a time or I get a flush on my hands and they itch, otherwise I've exhausted allergy reasons (other than nerves).—Mrs. M.P., Reedsport, Oregon.

A. It is obvious that you may have a fungus infection, but I would start a treatment program from a different approach. First, it seems that you are suffering from an A and D deficiency. I would use cod liver oil in rather large doses. Any toxicity found from A and D vitamins has always been caused by synthetic forms. The natural forms are nontoxic and large doses can be taken with impunity. The only possible exception is that large doses of oil could upset the gallbladder on occasion. Probably two tablespoonfuls at bedtime with a little orange juice would suffice. Maybe even more Vitamin A is needed here. Certainly 100,000 units daily for three months would be indicated before concluding that this would not correct the condition.

The next needed item is hydrochloric acid. It takes time to correct the HCl deficiency. I would give several tablets, even five after each meal. This certainly will be an overdosage sooner or later, but it then can be cut back. As your own body begins to secrete more HCl, the dosage needed in pill form can be reduced. Be wise and alert and you can solve some of your own problems.

You also mention symptoms strongly indicative of B-complex deficiency. Now the problem gets a bit ticklish. You should always take the whole B complex when taking a single B factor or vitamin. Brewer's yeast in liquid form is my favorite.* On top of this, you probably need more of the B-2 or riboflavin group. Your allergies will respond to *large* doses of pantothenic acid.

Local application of 10 percent gentian violet and acriflavin in saturated glycerin may help eradicate fungus infections involving the vaginal tract.

*See Product Information.

41. Strokes

Vitamins

Q. *My aunt, who is in her late 70s, had a light stroke not too long ago. She is in the hospital now. Her arm and leg are somewhat bad. In all books on health, strokes are listed along with heart trouble. Are they the same? I have read how good such vitamins as C, B, and E are in heart trouble. I would like to know if they would help in strokes?*—J.W., Kansas City, Missouri.

A. You are certainly correct, there is much good in Vitamins C, B and E for heart trouble. They are also useful in strokes and many other conditions. The only drawback I know of is in the use of Vitamin E which can and does sometimes cause high blood pressure to go higher. This is not always so, but is true part of the time. I would suggest starting with a lower dosage and gradually increasing it. If you stop using it, the amount of Vitamin E in the blood disappears within three days. So, even if trouble develops, the length of time involved is relatively short. Of course, a stroke can happen in an instant of time. A fairly safe dosage would be 100 I.U. three times daily for a month. If no results are forthcoming, the dosage can be increased. Continue until you find your correct dosage. If you are faced with an acute condition, then you must take some chances. Start with 100 I.U. three times daily, increase this until any symptoms seem to be improved. Every patient has his own dosage needs. You must find this.

One observation on DMSO was made when it was used on quadriplegics (all limbs paralyzed). In this instance all that was done was to paint the limbs with DMSO. Lo and behold, within two years of daily application some movement was seen.

Slight Stroke

Q. *I am 59, and I just recently suffered a slight stroke—blood pressure 180/90. For the last year I have been taking several natural food supplements. I have very few colds and my arthritis in the hips is better. But why the stroke?*—R.H., Calif.

A. A slight stroke probably means that there is a beginning blockage of one of the smaller arteries in the brain. This is probably due to the formation of hardened arteries and/or the increased viscosity of the blood. In the former situation the use of high dosages of Vitamin E, gradually increased so that the blood pressure does not rise, is good. It is also wise to take associated amounts of Vitamin C in large dosages. Lecithin helps to reduce the hardened arteries. The use of polyunsaturated fatty acids is important here since they tend to protect against the abnormal deposition of cholesterol and the triglycerides in arteries. Inositol as well as choline and methionine are very valuable in such conditions. Vitamins A and F also contribute to the mobilization of the abnormally deposited calcium. Liver stimulation with beet leaf juice tablets helps, too.

In the second condition, where the blood viscosity is increased so that clotting is enhanced, the use of orthophosphoric acid tends to thin the blood without the dangerous complication often found with the drug blood thinners.*

There are two things about the list of vitamin supplements you have given. One is that there are too many separate vitamins used, which means that they are not natural and balanced as in nature even though they may have been derived from natural sources. They are vitamins being used as drugs. The second is the use of dolomite. There is something about this preparation which actually impedes the proper absorption of calcium into the system. Otherwise, your thoughts are moving in the right direction.

*See Product Information.

Strokes

Q. *My husband has experienced a number of minor strokes. Could you tell us about strokes?*—Mrs. W.E.S., Melvindale, Michigan.

A. Your husband is a candidate for the EDTA therapy. This is a relatively new treatment where the chelation material is injected into the blood on a daily basis for some 20 days. The material chelates the calcium as well as other minerals in the blood stream and is taken out through the urine. The technique rids the body of excess calcium which has been deposited in places like arteries. A doctor who uses this technique must be chosen wisely for extensive experience, proper supervision and care of the patient undergoing it.

The diet should be mainly one of fresh, raw fruits, vegetables, nuts and seeds. Always avoid man-made foods. White flour, white sugar and white rice are the worst offenders.

He needs all the routine vitamins and minerals. Vitamin C and the bioflavonoids are extremely important.

Stroke

Q. *My mother died from a stroke at age 78. The stroke was due to hardening of the arteries. One doctor has told me this is hereditary. Could you please give me your opinion on this?*—Mr. J.O.Q., San Francisco, Ca.

A. Baloney! In a word. You have hardened arteries because of what you have been eating and metabolizing for the past 50 years or so. You may have certain congenital or cultural factors because you eat approximately what your mother used to eat, and still follow old habits. But it is your fault for having hardened arteries, not your mother's.

Nutritionally, you may use high Vitamin C, lecithin, B complex, E natural and avoid man-made fats. This is the nutritional approach to hardened arteries.

EDTA has come to the forefront in recent months as a means of softening hardened arteries and improving local circulation. I would certainly seriously consider its use here when the condition is very bad and desperate measures are needed to save life and function.

Possible Stroke

Q. *My 69-year-old mother suffered what probably was a stroke. There was never a clear-cut diagnosis made although she was seen and tested by 11 doctors—neurologists, neurosurgeons and throat specialists during a month-long stay in the hospital. Her throat and the left side of her face are the only areas affected by paralysis. She is being fed through a tube directly into the stomach. Although before she had this episode there was a good deal of stress, she had always been basically very active and in good health. She can now swallow tiny amounts of liquids, is alert and regaining strength. She is receiving many vitamin and mineral supplements via tube feeding including B and C.*—J.M., Montgomery, Ala.

A. One of the serious troubles with modern medicine is that there are too many specialists and consultants. The net result is, who is in charge? Who is the responsible one? I would certainly prefer the good old-fashioned country doctor. He may not have known as much, but he was responsible and did all he could to solve the problem at hand.

For strokes and other such problems, I refer my patients for EDTA therapy. This method helps soften hardened arteries and correct circulatory difficulties. There are several doctors throughout the country who are now doing this work.

The American Academy of Medical Preventics, 350 Parnassus, Suite 700, San Francisco, Cal. 94117, can advise you.

Peripheral Circulation

Q. *My sister's husband had a stroke. From his shoulder down to his right leg he is in a brace. My grandson has an ulcer at the age of 14. Is there anything you could suggest for him? I have trouble with arthritis in my hands, knee joints in both legs, and fingers. The pain is terrific. Can you suggest anything for the problems?*—H.R., Newbury, Wis.

A. I find it very difficult to answer questions like this. Mostly because there is so much to say that it would take volumes. Each case is different, unique, and needs different treatment. However, some things are basic to all. Among other things, the body needs to be fed properly. The veins carry the blood supply as well as remove the waste products. The circulatory system is of vital importance to health.

Have you ever wondered why when something happens healthwise to a person, there seem to be several things that happen at the same time? Could it be that there is some sort of common denominator to the whole situation? I believe there is, and that it is the circulatory system. If you have hardened arteries in one place, like the brain, and there is a stroke, it does not mean you have hardened arteries only in this one area. In fact, one should expect to find hardened arteries in many different areas—usually throughout the whole body. In this case, the brain arterial system has hardened ahead of the other areas of the body so that a stroke occurred. But this disturbance of balance in the brain caused other areas to fall below the critical level of circulatory integrity and the kidney, heart, pancreatic or any other area also became involved.

Since the arterial system plays a vital role in the function of *all* the other systems, it stands to reason that many diseases are related to deficient circulation in various local areas.

It has been rightly said that we die from the outside inward. When you begin to have circulation problems in the extremities, it is already a well-advanced situation throughout the body. Take heed. Take care of your peripheral circulation. Read up in nutrition books of all nutritional factors which affect the circulation: Vitamins E, A, B-6, lecithin and others.

42. Thyroid

Hyperthyroidism

Q. *What type of vitamins, minerals, or nutrition would you suggest for hyperthyroidism?*—F.D., Corvallis, Oregon.

A. I believe that a deficiency of iodine is the primary cause of hyperthyroidism. Paradoxically, both under- and overactive thyroid functions can be caused by deficiency of iodine. The type of reaction depends upon the individual. In one situation the deficiency of iodine causes the thyroid to decrease in function due to lack of raw materials from which to develop thyroxine.

In the other situation the thyroid reacts differently. The deficiency of iodine causes the thyroid to produce an insufficient quantity or a poor quality of thyroxine which then causes the responding organs to demand more and more thyroxine. More and more is produced but of less and poorer quality. The needs are not met but the toxicity of the thyroxine does not decrease, resulting in hyperthyroidism. This is an opinion based upon clinical reactions and not measurements in the laboratory. (Hyperthyroidism means overactive thyroid; hypothyroidism means underactive.)

Iodine Need

Q. *What do doctors who aren't interested in nutrition say is the minimum amount of iodine a person needs?*—J.S., Ontario, Canada.

A. Medically accepted standard for iodine needs in the human body is 3 micrograms per Kg weight or 200 micrograms for a 150-pound man. 200 micrograms is the same as 0.2 mg.

My opinion, based upon clinical experience, is that the average need is nearer to 1.0 mg daily.

Excessive Perspiration

Q. Ever since I can remember I have been plagued by excessive perspiration in the summertime, and even in the winter where the steam heated rooms are warm. It is extremely embarrassing because it is my face that perspires most, and I dread going anywhere in the summer months where there is no air conditioning. My health has always been good for the past few years. I've taken vitamin supplements and try to eat a wholesome diet. Can you suggest anything for this problem?—Mrs. F.M., Brooklyn, N.Y.

A. Excessive perspiration is a symptom suggestive of thyroid gland malfunction, something generally based upon the shortage of B complex in the system, plus the probable shortage of iodine. In most diets consumed in the country today, one can easily find a shortage of B vitamins. In addition to the B vitamins, I would suggest a trial of kelp to increase the iodine supply for your thyroid. I am not sure that iodized salt will supply the needs here, but certainly uniodized salt would not.

I have also used half tincture of iodine and half water, 1 drop daily on food or in water. This is a simple source of about 1.0 mg iodine per drop.

Underactive Thyroid

Q. A year ago I came down with a severe case of serum hepatitis. Since then I have been taking three One-A-Day vitamins (two regular and one with iron), Vitamin B complex with Vitamin C, 1200 I.U. of Vitamin E and B-12 shots once or twice a week. After a year of this regimen with no improvement, my doctor ran some more tests and found that I have an underactive thyroid. For several weeks now I have been taking pills for the thyroid which are supposed to give me energy, but have not.

I would like to know two things: What do you think about the assortment of vitamins I'm taking? And is it pos-

sible that the Vitamin E is cancelling out the effects of the thyroid pills?—V.S., Staten Island, New York.

A. I really do not think too much of your selection of vitamins. You have fallen into the trap: synthetic vitamins on the label do not give the results of the natural vitamins in the stomach. Natural and organic preparations supposedly contain all the naturally associated synergistic micronutrients necessary for the vitamins to work. It is necessary to take minerals and enzymes too and eat balanced meals of naturally raised foods.

Insofar as your thyroid problem is concerned, I don't think that Vitamin E cancels out the activity of the thyroid substance. It would be necessary to know how much you are taking of the thyroid preparation and which one. Thyroid should be adjusted upward in dosage, on a monthly basis, until an overdosage is detected—then cut down. I use pork thyroid because it is closer to the hormone composition of the human thyroid. Beef thyroid is quite dissimilar.

Iodine intake is important too. I use one drop of half water, half tincture of iodine each day. This would be about 1 mg, which is almost a universal dosage.

Underactive Thyroid

Q. *I've been told that underactivity of the thyroid gland in women is not uncommon. I have this problem. What causes this problem and what vitamins, minerals, etc., might help? What does cytomel do for it?*—Mrs. L.B.M., Denver, Colorado.

A. Let's just say that underactive thyroid is common in both men and women. It may be a little more noticeable in women because they usually come for attention a little sooner than men. The condition is one where there are insufficient amounts of thyroxin secreted by the thyroid gland. Thus the metabolic rate of the individual is reduced a bit and all sorts of subnormal activity results. Some of the obvious clinical syndromes are: overweight, dysmenorrhea, laziness, fatigue, a need for too much sleep, low blood pressure, etc., etc.

In studying this condition, the researchers have discovered that a type of goiter develops quite frequently in certain geographical areas, such as around the Great Lakes, the Pacific Northwest and other smaller areas. They also discovered that the incidence of this condition was greatly lessened by the consumption of iodized salt. (Nowadays, it is becoming unpopular to use iodized salt, so the incidence of goiter is again increasing.) In other words, the causative factor thus revealed is the lack of iodine in the diet.

The mechanism of this process goes something like this: The body demands thyroxin for proper action. The thyroid responds by secreting thyroxin. If the thyroxin is not adequately available because of lack of iodine, then either a reduced amount of thyroxin is secreted or a low quality thyroxin is secreted. This deficiency does not solve the need of the tissues so the demand is still being made upon the brain to cause more secretion. Now, either of two things may happen. First, the thyroid can secrete more and more of the poor quality thyroxin which could still contain the elements to cause nervousness, etc., and a toxic thyroid could develop. Or, the thyroid could become exhausted in its effort to supply the need and fail to respond effectively. This would result in the underactive thyroid. Both of these conditions are caused by lack of iodine in the diet.

The item which could be of the greatest value in controlling this condition would be kelp. Kelp is a wonderful substance containing the concentration of all the minerals found in the sea water. The iodine concentration is especially high in kelp. Or one could take half water, half tincture of iodine, *one drop daily*.

Goiter Operation

Q. *I am concerned about my husband's health. He had a goiter operation. His health improved until about five years ago when he had a stroke which affected his sight. Diabetes set in, as well as high blood pressure and heart trouble. The doctors have him on thyroid pills, blood pressure pills and diabetes tablets. He weighs more than 200 and can hardly get his clothes on. Is there any help for him through vitamins and health foods?*—H. R., Howard Lake, Minn.

A. Here is a sad tale of woe which is so common today, due to two basic factors. One is poor delivery of blood to the areas involved, actually the whole body; and second, poor removal of waste products of metabolism from the cellular level via the lymph system. This man needs a total body-cleansing program plus other health measures: rest, exercise, physiotherapy, diet, massage, manipulations and anything else which will tend to help the individual cells work more normally. This man is probably so full of toxic metabolic waste products that I fear the damage may not be repairable. Proper treatment for this condition should have started 20 years ago.

He also needs medical expertise in management of his thyroid problem.

43. Varicose Veins

Enlarged Veins

Q. *What causes enlarged veins on the lower arms and hands and what can be done to make them disappear?*—P.J., Colon, Republic of Panama.

A. In my opinion, venous congestion in any part of the body is an indication of liver congestion. The congestion of the liver may not have progressed to the stage of cirrhosis or hepatitis but these conditions are in the offing. My first approach is to detoxify the liver and to supply the nutrients which are especially favorable to good liver function. B complex is, of course, primary. However, it must be a basic natural form and not a conglomeration of synthetic multiple vitamin formulas. Yeast and liver are good sources. Moreover, liver tissue is very valuable in treatment. Large doses of Vitamin C are indicated, too. Collinsonia root tablets help dilated veins.*

Dilated Blood Vessels

Q. *Do you have any information on the causes of dilated blood vessels?*—J.C., Alexandria, Virginia.

A. Dilated blood vessels could be dilated arteries, veins or capillaries. I presume you are not talking about aneurisms. Dilated capillaries and veins could be caused by liver malfunction and congestion. This is usual. In fact, I always look for these as telltale evidence of liver malfunction. Also, naturally, the dilated veins could be caused by some sort of block to the free flow of blood back to the heart.

You mention the possibility of an allergic reaction causing this problem. This could be true. To make a guess as to the cause would be foolhardy since so many things

*See Product Information.

355

could cause the reaction. It depends upon you as to which one. Nicotinic acid, one of the B complex, can cause dilation of the capillary bed, but I do not think you mean this type.

Varicose Veins

Q. *I am 44 years old and have noticed that within the last year I have many spider type veins in my legs and am worried about having varicose veins. I take several supplements and also try to eat as much health food as possible. I would like to know if anything can be done through nutrition to help this situation?*—J.G., Ohio.

A. The commonest remedy for varicose veins is Vitamin E. It is necessary to take large enough doses. Strangely enough, it seems that it takes larger doses to accomplish the same results than it did a decade ago. Dr. Shute has positive evidence in his files that the content of Vitamin E in many Vitamin E products today is less than the dosage stated on the label. This is a sad affair.

The second vitamin of vital importance in varicose veins is Vitamin B complex. The integrity of the veins is maintained by this vitamin complex. Vitamin C, particularly the bioflavonoids, plays a part also.

In the herb line, collinsonia root is a good remedy for varicose veins.

Hemorrhoids

Q. *I started on health foods 18 months ago, and shortly thereafter had my first case of hemorrhoids. They have continued about every four months since then. My proctologist has no answer for their appearance as I am under no tension. He did suggest that perhaps there is an allergy to wheat or brewer's yeast.*—P.C., Los Angeles, California.

A. I am sure your better diet did not cause the hemorrhoids. Neither does tension. Hemorrhoids are the result of poor liver function and/or poor structure of the hemorrhoidal veins. At least, when one develops hemorrhoids the suspected problem is liver trouble until proven wrong. Do not be too hasty to accept the fact that the liver is not at fault because the methods of measuring liver function are often misleading.

Allergy to brewer's yeast is a shot in the dark. Even if you were allergic to wheat or brewer's yeast, the chance of your developing hemorrhoids from it is so slim that the odds would be one in a trillion.

Actually, brewer's yeast and wheat tend to strengthen venous structures so that hemorrhoidal dilation could be reduced and vein structure improved.

44. Vitamins

Food Supplementation

Q. *A friend of mine, well versed in food supplementation, tells people they should take food supplements for at least four months before judging whether or not they are benefiting from them. His explanation for this is that the blood renews itself every four months. Is this true?*

He also maintains that if you get a bad reaction—constipation, nausea, or whatever—upon starting a supplementation program, you should increase your dosage so that the body adjusts more quickly to the improved nutrition. I always thought it better to reduce your dosage and build up gradually. What is your opinion?—P.S., Brea, California.

A. I do not know whether the blood entirely renews itself within four months. It is true that the average lifetime of the red cells is about 120 days, however. The life of other factors is from three days to ten weeks.

When you develop symptoms from a nutritional detoxification program, are you supposed to push your luck or back down and allow the body to react more slowly and comfortably? I am sure that this is the point of "art" in medicine. When do you push and when do you retreat? Unfortunately, I cannot give you a pat answer. My usual approach is to give moral support to the wavering patient who is having difficulties which I think will blow over soon and rather easily. For example, I find that most of the detoxification symptoms occur during the stringent mono or duo diet time. When this occurs the simple addition of one avocado per day to the diet is usually enough to slow down the action so that the patient gets relief but does not lose the effects of the program. If not exact, the 120 days is practical.

Natural vs. Synthetic

Q. *I take Vitamin B complex. Also I have tried brewer's yeast, but can't stand the taste. My arms and shoulders ached so bad that I couldn't sleep nights. I haven't taken any B for several days and the aches are fast leaving me. Can you figure what is wrong?*—Mrs. E.H., Independence, Missouri.

A. I do believe that you are taking synthetic vitamins. This, in itself, is enough reason to expect some complications. Synthetics are certainly not the same as the natural. For instance, Vitamin C is usually one factor only in ascorbic acid, yet there are some five different elements which make up the whole natural Vitamin C complex, plus certain naturally associated products. Also, brewer's yeast is not the same as produced by all companies. The flake form is more palatable and can be taken in juices of your choice.

Multivitamin Potency

Q. *I am wondering whether potencies of multivitamins and minerals are sufficient when compacted in such a little capsule or tablet? Can the minimum daily requirement for the body be met? Or must I take multivitamin and mineral supplements plus other vitamins separately?*—V.R., Kaiser Dededo, Guam.

A. To answer this question a few words must be said about tablet and capsule production. First, let me say that it is impossible to make a high potency tablet from natural factors. If all the naturally associated micronutrients were to be included in the preparation, a high potency tablet would be so large it could not be swallowed. If you will check all labels now, you will see that the wording reveals this, for example, "Vitamin C from rose hips and ascorbic acid." This does not say that all the Vitamin C is from rose hips. The same applies to B complex vitamins and E and the rest of them; the labeling is deceptive. They do not contain the naturally associated micronutrients which are important for life.

MDR

Q. *I have heard that some oil-soluble vitamins, such as A and D, can be toxic to the liver and other organs if taken in large overdoses. Yet my own choice of multivitamins, like many others, contains as much as 625 percent of the MDR for these and other vitamins.*

If overdoses can cause liver toxicity and other ailments, why are they included in such large amounts in these products?—Mr. M.B.C., Dallas, Texas.

A. MDR is simple *Minimum* Daily Requirements—and that is exactly what it is. It is nowhere near optimal daily requirements or any other sort of level. Do not be fooled by these words. Your normal average daily needs may be many hundreds of times the MDR. You are unique and your needs are yours alone. It is my opinion, based upon years of nutritional practice of medicine, that there are no overdosages on *natural* vitamins. It is always the synthetics taken in large doses which become toxic on occasion. Possibly, if you already have liver disease, large doses of oil of any type could cause a reaction. This is because of the oil content or rancidity, and not because of the vitamin content.

Vitamin Poisoning

Q. *I started using Vitamin C (rosehips + bioflavonoids) some time ago for about four months, noticing only slightly higher resistance to colds. Then I read an article in some magazine (not a health magazine) about the possibility of vitamin poisoning and discontinued use. Recently, someone advised me to take Vitamin C for a cold and I told her about my experience with Vitamin C. She informed me the article was untrue as the body does not store Vitamin C—if there is excess, it is expelled. Do you agree with this?*—M.S., Montreal, Canada.

A. The so-called vitamin poisoning scare you read about was started against the findings of Linus Pauling, the noted Nobel Prize winner. The orthodox medical establishment and drug firms were (and are) fighting desperately to find some sort of defense. In my experience, it is practically impossible to cause Vitamin C poisoning, even with the use of the synthetic variety. Large dosages of Vitamin C *may* cause excessive gas, but this can be relieved by chewing the tablets or by taking C in powdered form.

Hypervitaminosis A

Q. *I went to a doctor who gave me 50,000 units of A—shot in the hip when I had asked for a calcium shot. He said A was better for my aching tired bones. He already knew I was on carrot juice so why he insisted on A, I will never know. This "A" shot which was given to me almost seven weeks ago had the worst possible effect on my body. Bone, ligaments and cell pain almost to the point of drug taking. Arthritis and pain are now in my hips, spine, knees and ankles. What would you suggest to counteract this toxic A?*—H.A., Los Angeles, Ca.

A. Hypervitaminosis A can occur in humans. The reaction usually occurs six to fifteen months after onset of starting excessive dosages of the vitamin. The symptoms consist of hard, tender lumps in the extremities and cortical thickening of underlying bones. Additional findings in some patients include fissures of the lips, loss of hair, dry skin, jaundice and hepatomegaly (enlarged liver). The clinical symptoms usually subside 72 hours after withdrawing the excessive intake. The blood levels fall in six weeks and cortical hyperostoses are gradually and slowly resorbed over a period of several months.

It does not sound as if you suffer from too much A. It is much more likely that you suffer from an allergic reaction to the injection. All injections, except for a very few very special ones, contain preservatives. These chemicals often are the cause of the reactions but are not considered in the clinical situation at first. Chemicals are very important and can be the cause of much suffering and are often overlooked.

In the clinical approach to your problem, I would first consider large dosages of Vitamin C. This is a fantastic

cleanser and antiallergic remedy. The next approach
would be to enhance liver function. Any sort of liver detoxification program would help. Then, of course, you
need general rebuilding of the body. Detoxification comes
first, then rebuilding the body, in this order.

Vitamin E

Q. *You discussed Vitamin E complex or mixed with tocopherols derived from the so-called natural sources, including the four types of tocopherols which contain all the
naturally occurring synergistic factors. What are the problems connected with taking Vitamin E only in the form of
alpha tocopherol? How does one get a prescribed dosage
of alpha tocopherol in changing over to the E complex?*—
M.H., Cincinnati, O.

A. Many Vitamin E preparations are mixed tocopherols
and are rated in terms of d-alpha only. In other words 100
I.U. would mean 100 units of d-alpha and the other tocopherols are added. The disadvantage of taking d-alpha
only as compared to the total complex is probably more
theoretical than real. The pure d-alpha does not contain
the naturally associated micronutrients and, as such, there
will be a shortage of these particular items, although at
present it is hard to pinpoint symptoms of this deficiency.

It is similar to the Vitamin C complex. Ascorbic acid is
the one factor most publicized and perhaps most useful
for certain conditions. It is, however, only one part of a
whole complex group or family of related factors which
go to make up the total Vitamin C complex. The whole is
always better than one part. For example, I have never
been able to cure pyorrhea with ascorbic acid, but can do
so with the natural C products or bioflavonoids. So, though
not yet proved, the whole Vitamin E complex must have
more power than just the one factor d-alpha tocopherol.
Wheat germ oil is natural Vitamin E.

Vitamin B Deficiency

Q. *I have a problem with my tongue. I understand that this condition of the tongue can indicate a severe Vitamin B deficiency. Although my tongue is rarely sensitive and only once have I seen even a trace of blood at one of the creases, I believe that I take (with my doctor's approval) far more than normal requirements of B. I suspect malabsorption rather than inadequacy. Can you suggest anything?*—C.W., Albuquerque, New Mexico.

A. What you describe certainly is a B complex deficiency, at least until definitely proven to be something else. First, you must throw out the concept of minimal daily requirements. This may be okay, though I doubt it, for the average person—whoever he is—but it certainly is not enough for you. Your requirements for B complex must be fantastic. True, a part of the problem may be in absorption, but it sounds like your requirements are just plain high. Brewer's yeast is a good place to start. Take as much as your system will tolerate. Then add to the program other types of natural B complex. Liver and wheat germ are good sources. Then add the tablet supplements, trying to stick to the natural ones.

In order to maximize the digestion and absorption, you need a thorough bowel cleansing program. This means cleansing, plus installation of beneficial organisms conducive to the growth of the acidophilus organisms. This is a must because these organisms actually do produce some of the B complex as well as aid in the absorption of such. Yogurt or Kafir and acidophilus cultures can help.

B Complex Deficiency

Q. *My sister has had a sore mouth for over a year. Nothing has helped. She has been to many doctors, and specialists; she has taken B-12 shots and all kinds of vitamins. For a month now she has been taking brewer's yeast, rice polishings and lecithin mixed in her blender but* *her mouth is not better. Could you suggest anything?*— A.P., Englewood, Florida.

A. The sore mouth syndrome is probably a B complex deficiency. In this case, it could easily be because the absorption is poor. Apparently, the intake of these vitamins is more than adequate, so it must be that she is not digesting or absorbing them. I cannot tell from this distance, but I would guess that she lacks hydrochloric acid. Her condition might be solved by the use of apple cider vinegar, but the hydrochloric acid is more sure.

Folic Acid

Q. *I have a grayish brown skin pigmentation which is called "pregnancy cap" by Adelle Davis. This developed while taking oral contraceptives. I am not pregnant. She says it disappears when five milligrams of folic acid are taken after each meal. I got the folic acid from Canada and began taking it. After about five or six days I was constipated and had to stop taking it. Also my stool had turned black. I am not taking any other medication or vitamins.*

Can you tell me what else I must be taking in order to take that much folic acid for a few weeks?—M.S., Berkeley, California.

A. You are apparently a good example of why the FDA put the ban on folic acid. You are always supposed to take it with B-12. However, that is not your problem here.

Out of the clear blue, you started taking folic acid. Folic acid is a good cleanser of the system and, apparently, it has worked in your case. I would simply suggest that you start taking it in smaller doses and gradually increase the dosage. You should also take all the B complex at the same time. This can be accomplished in the form of liver and yeast.

Vitamin B-15

Q. *In a previous column you mentioned pangamic acid, Vitamin B-15. I note it is for sale in Germany. Could you explain how I could purchase this Vitamin B-15?*

A. Vitamin B-15 is not generally available in the United States. Vitamin B-15 or pangamic acid is naturally found in seeds. It was discovered in apricot kernels, but is found in all sorts of seeds. For this reason, one should always eat seeds of any fruit eaten.

Vitamin C

Q. *My husband has been taking Vitamin C tablets (mostly acerola, cherry and rose hips) for nearly a year, using about 2,400 mg daily. He took them to control asthma which he developed several years ago at the age of 56. He had taken allergy shots which did not seem to help much and allergy capsules caused prostate trouble. We then became aware of health foods and vitamins, and much to our delight discovered that Vitamin C helped tremendously.*

However, about eight months after starting the Vitamin C, my husband started having trouble with urinary bladder stones. He had them removed about one month ago. They were in all sizes with the largest being ⅘-inch in diameter. They were diagnosed as being uric acid stones and the doctor says that they were caused by the Vitamin C, and that he must stop taking them at once. He was also told to take citrocarbonate, an antacid, to counteract the acid in his body.—Mrs. C.H., Defiance, Ohio.

A. Offhand, uric acid crystals are deposited in the urinary system primarily because of insufficient liver action in cleansing the system of uric acid. Vitamin C has no effect in this area to the best of my knowledge. In actuality, Vitamin C is a good liver stimulant so should cut down on the chances of stone formation. In addition to the Vitamin

C for the asthma, why doesn't your husband try taking large doses of pantothenic acid for allergy—like 1000 mg four times daily?

Too Many Vitamins?

Q. *I would like you to comment on the following statement: "Long term use of vitamins weakens the body's ability to absorb vitamins from food and to manufacture vitamins within the body.*"—Mrs. M.K.S., Menlo Park, California.

A. In this connection, I have to know what kind of vitamins. If they are using the high concentration, synthetic variety, I would thoroughly agree. In fact, these items should not be used as dietary supplements in the first place. If they are talking about the high potency natural and organic vitamins usually found in the health food stores, I would not be so much concerned. The key point is this: If the natural and organic vitamins in the truest sense are used, there need be no concern about taking them for too long a period of time. These items are simply concentrated food substances. That is to say, food that has had the water removed. Once in a great while I do find that a patient going through my intensive therapeutic nutritional program indicates that too much is being taken into the system and a rest period is needed. But this occurs only when large dosages of the supplements are taken over a long period of time. In reality, it becomes a situation where there is too rapid detoxification for the excretory organs to handle.

Regarding Brand Names

Q. *Congratulations on your new book,* A New Breed of Doctor. *It is terrific and very practical, too. However, I wish to know why you mention brand names of products you use. Some of these cannot be found in health food stores. I think it is very unfair of you to do such a thing.*—L.B., Carmel, California.

VITAMINS 367

A. Yes, I mention brand names of products which I use for a very practical reason. When I first was beginning to test nutritional methods, I used products which did not do the job desired and almost tossed the whole idea out the window. Fortunately, I did come in contact with a good product, almost by accident, so that I really could see that there was value therein. Later I found others which were also very helpful.

Again, if I did not state brand names of products I use, other doctors who might be influenced by my ideas could possibly try products which might be inferior and not get results desired. Thus, the whole nutritional effort would be given a black eye because of some poor quality item used in place of a good one. My list of products contains only the ones I know and, yet, there are many more which I am sure exist but that I just do not know personally. Thus, I feel obligated to mention those I do know.

Actually, some of the products I mentioned are available only through your doctor, whether he be M.D., D.O., N.D., D.V.M., D.D.S., or D.C. Thus, I would encourage you to take my book to your doctor to encourage him to become aware of nutritional power by getting him to order these products for you and to follow your progress. Naturally, these items are derived from natural foods and held in the highest esteem in nutritional circles.

Last but not least, you apparently did not check all the items which I use since there are several brands available in the health food stores.

45. Weight Problems

Sugar Craving

Q. *I have always had a weight problem. As of late last year, I completely gave up drinking alcohol. However, as a result, a never-ending craving for chocolate and sweets has developed, which I never had before. What food element is in both alcohol and sweets that can be supplied through a particular food supplement pill or health food that will end this craving? I get sugar in coffee, eat lots of fruits, take a wheat germ, Vitamin B-6 and a mineral tablet.*—E.D., Atlanta, Georgia.

A. This letter represents the lack of knowledge that exists in the United States today due to lack of adequate and proper nutritional education. Many admit that alcohol is not good for the individual and that it is bad to gain so much weight. However, the widespread habit of taking both coffee and sugar is appalling! I personally think that coffee and sugar are causing more trouble in this country than alcohol, and I do not belittle the alcohol problem either. The results of sugar metabolism are completely misunderstood. I have many patients who suffer from low blood sugar, who have been advised by their own doctors to simply eat a candy bar when they have the symptoms. This is the very thing that will make the problem worse, since a great number of hypoglycemic cases are caused by eating sugar.

Just stop a moment and think what the usual American eats during the day. A cup of coffee with sugar for breakfast, which causes a quick rise in the blood sugar, and because the pancreas assumes a big meal is coming along, it produces too much insulin and causes the elevated blood sugar to come down again in a hurry. Adding a sweet roll or white toast or cold cereal only compounds the rise and fall of the blood sugar level. A cigarette helps the blood sugar to go up and then allows it to drop again. At coffee break, another cup with sugar and a donut results in another quick rise and fall of blood sugar. Lunch may include a sandwich of white bread and meat preparation. Bread is no better than sugar in coffee and the meat preparation probably contains sugar, also. Then top it off with a piece of pie, plus a cigarette. At two o'clock, it is time for a soft drink, usually one with caffein, and more cigarettes. This effect lasts for a couple of hours, until time for a late afternoon cup of coffee. Supper is not much better. Instant potatoes, white bread, frankfurters and the dessert all contain large amounts of sugar. Do you realize that sugar is consumed at the rate of two pounds per week by everyone in the USA today?.

The "food element" common to both chocolate and alcohol is sugar; the effect on the pancreas is the same. Both sugar and alcohol create a craving for more. The opposite is also true; the less you take, the less you want, though you may have to taper off gradually.

Now, what *should* you eat? Two weeks on a grapefruit and celery diet, followed by a completely raw diet for a month will work wonders. You should be observed by a specialist during this time and also continue with all the supplements.

From then on, the diet needed is a high natural carbohydrate, moderate protein one with plenty of fats, especially the polyunsaturates. There should be a goodly amount of nonprocessed or natural carbohydrates, especially the low carbohydrate vegetables. And supplements should not be limited to one or two, *but all the vitamins and minerals in natural form*. Your diet has evidently been depleted for so long, you need everything available for compensation.

Underweight Problems

Q. *I have been extremely thin all my life and would like to know of any suggestions you might have in regard to gaining weight?*—C.L., Glendale, California.

A. Barring the possibilities that the problem lies in either heredity or psychological factors, the first thing to do is outline the best type of basic nutritional program you can. This means there must be an abundance of organically grown foods, wholesomely prepared and the intake of the necessary food supplements. Oils are needed so the function of the liver and pancreas can be maintained at normal or better. There is no easy way to gain weight. It is a matter of a goodly amount of the best foods in conjunction with the supplements and digestion aids needed to do the job. The latter may be the hidden factor which will turn the tide for you.

Overweight Problems

Q. *Every time I try to lose weight I get sick. Last time, a month or so ago, I had pneumonia. I've been to doctors and all they want to do is give me diet pills to appease the appetite I don't have and water pills that make me ill. Could you please help me?*—D.S., Yucaipa, California.

A. The problem of losing weight is one that has been hashed and rehashed. It may be glandular in origin, or a form of malnutrition where one item may be in short supply so that the person has the desire to eat more to get that item he craves. It may also be a matter of mineral balance. In some, it is due to a long intestinal tract so that more of the food eaten is absorbed than normal (or slow peristalsis will do the same). All in all, it is really a compound problem.

Recently, I have devised a program which seems to be promising. It consists of a bowel-cleansing program, using a gelatinous material* for a period of five days. The first three days are on fruit and vegetable juices with water only, and six servings of the gelatinous material. The next two days are on a raw fruit and vegetable diet with three servings of the gelatinous material. The next several days up to 14 are on an 80 percent raw diet and one serving of the gelatinous material. Then this routine is repeated each month until the desired weight is obtained. Of course, one must not go crazy over food on the two weeks between

*See Product Information.

sessions, but one can be fairly "normal." After the first five days, the menu is supplemented with certain vitamins and minerals and hydrochloric acid to aid digestion.

I abhor the use of the diet pills to curb appetite. They never seem to accomplish the aim. They simply stimulate the metabolism so that the calories are used up faster, still leaving overweight in their wake, or a resumption of former levels.

46. Product Information

I choose certain brands of products because I have found them helpful for patients. But, because of ethical and legal technicalities, I cannot mention the brand names of these products in this book. Otherwise the book would be charged with being a "commercial" for these products, which it is not. Or the FDA can construe that the book is guilty of "labeling"—considered an illegal practice.

If you wish a product name, please send me a 3x5 card which includes the product identification, including the page number of the book where it is mentioned (I have more than one book). Please also include your name and address. Send a separate card for each product. I will relay these cards to the product distributor who will contact you directly. He cannot mention my name, so please be on the alert for the information.

47. Index

373